To: Susan and Carine
Many blessings

Bless My Bones
Why Calcium Doesn't Work
By Gene Ladd

Copyright 2008

Published by
Pleasant Stone Farm, Ltd.

ISBN #1-4392-1009-8

D0839142

TABLE OF CONTENTS

DEDICATION

To the memory of Granny Love, Matriarch of the Love family of Oteen, North Carolina and my late mother-in-law, Milica Maglica from Zlarin, an island off the Dalmatian coast of Croatia.

THE HUMP

Granny Love was my first best friend in life, the first person I remember outside of my immediate family to show and accept love. It was 1938, or perhaps 1939. I was born in 1935, and I am sharing some of my earliest memories with you. My parents rented an apartment in one of several houses on the Love family farm. Each morning when I went out to play, I would soon be knocking on the kitchen door at Granny Love's house. I was greeted with a loving hug and a voice that still reminds me of birds singing early in the morning. Always the greeting, "Bless my bones, look who it is". She would go to the warmer above her wood fired cook stove and take out a biscuit, still fresh from breakfast. She filled it with one of her homemade jams or jellies. Usually apple jelly, but sometimes she shared her black cherry jam with her young neighbor. She was a small woman, so small that I did not think of her as an adult. She was more like a fairy tale character. I recently learned that it was Granny Love's skill with home remedies that saved my life when whooping cough was killing hundreds of babies during an epidemic in our region.

In addition to being short, Granny Love was doubled over with a pronounced hump in her back. I wish I could have "blessed her bones". She had many sons and daughters and a large family of grandchildren and great grandchildren, plus many surrogates such as me. We lived in that apartment for a couple of years before moving to our own place not far away. I remember seeing many women with the hump in their back as I grew up in the mountains of Western North Carolina. I am sure we have all known women with the hump at one time or another. It amazes me that 70 years after those very special visits with my first best friend, Granny Loves everywhere still have very little available to them to avoid the disfigurement of osteoporosis.

That includes my mother-in-law. Milica Maglica was a statuesque and beautiful woman. When I first met her as a nervous suitor dating her daughter, Lillian, she was nearly six feet tall. She developed osteoporosis in her late seventies. She survived two classic hip breaks and lived to be ninety-two. As her spine collapsed and crumbled she developed a pronounced Dowager's hump and lost a full foot in height. Her heart was strong and she had better cholesterol readings than any of us, but the heart and lungs could not take the pressure created by the collapse of her spine.

Because of these two women who were very close to me, I was sensitive to the customers who came to me terrorized by their diagnosis of osteopenia or osteoporosis. The one thing they all feared was developing their grandmother's hump.

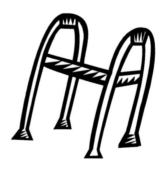

. <anatomy> The hard, calcified tissue of the skeleton of vertebrate animals, consisting very largely of calcic carbonate, calcic phosphate, and gelatin; as, blood and bone.

Even in the hardest parts of bone there are many minute cavities containing living matter and connected by minute canals, some of which connect with larger canals through which blood vessels ramify.

2. One of the pieces or parts of an animal skeleton; as, a rib or a thigh bone; a bone of the arm or leg; also, any fragment of bony substance. The frame or skeleton of the body.

Source:
Websters
Dictionary

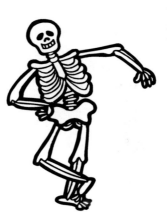

Usually when we encounter bones we see a hard piece of dead matter. It is what is left from the holiday ham or last night's chicken. Our grandparents had the good wisdom to boil the bones to extract some vital nutrients missing from our modern diets. Glucosamine and chondroitin sulfate, for example, were once plentiful in the American diet from soup bones. Today we have to supplement these nutrients for our arthritic joints. We all have a concept of the skeleton from Halloween or a horror movie. One might think of the skeleton as being connected, "toe bone to foot bone" or "foot bone to ankle bone". Our skeleton is very important for standing, walking and moving about, but this is only a small part of the contribution made to our well being by our bones. Actually, the bones that make up our skeleton are part of a multifunctioning vital organ. Healthy bones are important for much more than our mobility, and the risks from infirmed or malnourished bones are far more than bone break and falling.

Our skeleton houses the bone marrow. Healthy marrow is needed for healthy blood. The marrow is the place where our DNA is monitored and controlled. It is the source of the various response elements of our immune system. There is no single organ of the human body that can be called the immune organ housing the immune system. The marrow, however, comes very close. It is in this spongy material that fills the hallow space in the center of our bones that makes and releases the cells that are a major part of our immune response system.

If we do not have healthy bones, all of these functions can suffer. Our bones are also our mineral reserve or storage system. Our bodies can pull calcium and other minerals from our bones to maintain a balance among minerals. We also leach calcium from our bones to control the pH balance of our blood.

When our blood starts to become too acidic we release

calcium as an alkalizing agent. Our bodies function optimally with an acid/alkaline reading of 7.2 on a scale of zero to 14. The higher the acid in our blood, the lower the oxygen level. Lower levels of oxygen lead to heart disease, cancer and stress to every cell of the body. Later we will show how a high acid diet can be a leading cause of osteoporosis and low bone mass. We are constantly losing bone mass as we control the pH of our blood and maintain a balance among minerals in our body. If we are healthy and consuming the proper foods we will replace the bone mass as easily as we give it up. If we are giving up more than we are replacing, then we face the condition of osteoporosis from normal bone loss.

Volumes can be written on the importance of our bones for functions other than skeletal support. In this work, however, we will focus on osteoporosis, proper nourishment and supplements. There are many diseases and infirmities that can cause bone loss or poor bone quality. These conditions can be related to hormonal imbalance or the malfunction of various organs. I have no credentials to discuss these conditions. This book, therefore, focuses on bone health as it relates to nutrition.

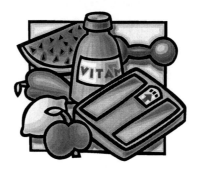

50/50?

I am sure by now you have heard that every woman in the United States has a 50/50 chance of experiencing a broken bone at least once in her lifetime after reaching the age of 50. One in two women are turning up in emergency rooms with broken bones in this broad age group, but to claim that all broken bones are caused by osteoporosis is misleading. It is important to know whether the person fell and broke a bone, or whether the bone break actually caused the fall.

Falls resulting in bone breaks are caused by poor eyesight, throw rugs, toys, pets, medications or combinations of medications that cause dizziness, unstable footwear, slippery conditions, inadequate lighting and scores of other normal household conditions. The classic bone break from osteoporosis is caused by weight stress on an eroded femur near the hip joint. In this case the bone breaks and the person falls from the lack of support. In the cases in which the person simply falls, the break may be caused by the severity of the impact more than by the condition of the bone. However, the condition of the bone will be a determining factor in the ability to survive the stress of the fall without breaking. All factors contribute to the 50/50 prediction.

There are several widespread misconceptions involving osteoporosis and bone mass. First we must point out that the people with the most bone mass are frequently more prone to bone break because of the quality of the bone matrix. A reduction of bone mass for people over fifty is a natural occurrence, and does not always mean their bones are more fragile. Asian women for example, with thin bones, do not experience the same rate of bone break as women in areas of the world where thicker bone mass is prevalent. We will address this phenomenon.

Recent scientific data emphasizes the importance of vitamin D3 in maintaining healthy bone mass. We can get only a small amount of this vitamin from food, and our most dependable supply comes from photosynthesis in sunlight. Our bodies make vitamin D3 from cholesterol in sunlight. It only takes a few minutes in the sun several times per week, but that becomes difficult in some zones of the Earth. Lifestyle demands also tend to limit the amount of time spent outdoors. Those with the darker skin pigments need more sunlight to produce vitamin D3. The widespread use of sunscreen creams also reduces the body's ability to make the vitamin. People who live in climate zones where sunlight is limited during the winter months can experience bone loss from a lack of vitamin D3. If we do not supplement vitamin D3 during periods in which we do not have sun exposure, we can have a serious deficiency. We need this important vitamin for much more than maintaining good bone mass. Vitamin D3 converts to essential hormones, and it is also important for cancer protection and an active immune response system. Several studies of geriatric Americans showed that most were deficient in vitamin D.

In the pages ahead, I will depend on scores of scientific studies for the information we will share. I will also draw on my own experience as a nutritional consultant to hundreds of women and men who were customers of my health food store over a period of nearly ten years. I have found that sharing actual real life experiences can be the best teacher. There are many convictions that cannot be supported by existing scientific studies, but we can know what we know from experience without "scientific" proof. Sometimes we must realize that prevailing scientific convictions often lag behind cutting edge reality by many years. Science itself can be overshadowed by convictions based on theories that should be replaced by up to date, proven studies. Pure science has no hesitation to embrace emerging truths. Commercial interests that claim a scientific platform on the other hand depend on confusion and doubt to protect their market shares. In life there is more mystery than knowledge. Those who have the courage to embrace the mysterious with faith and to trust their own experiences and instincts will not be lost in the arrogance of inadequate scientific measurements.

There are many things in life that we cannot perceive with our senses: touch, smell, taste, sound or sight. We cannot see time, but we can save it, spend it or waste it. We cannot see gravity, but we learn to respect it and co-operate with it at an early age. We cannot see energy, but we can use it. Faith is a form of energy. We are told that faith is part of imagination and without substance, part of a myth. To a degree gravity falls into the category of myth. Did an apple really fall from the tree hitting Isaac Newton on the head leading him to the discovery of gravity? Then gravity as we know it grew from a mythological story. We have developed formulas in physics that prove the existence of gravity and its constant characteristics. Who is to say that we could not develop similar science around faith, if we gave it the same attention we have given to gravity? If we do not co-operate with gravity we can fall. I submit that if we try to live our life without faith, we also stumble and fall.

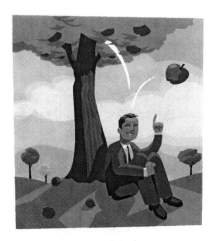

René Descartes (1596-1650) is one of the most important Western philosophers of the past few centuries. During his lifetime, Descartes was just as famous as an original physicist, physiologist and mathematician. But it is as a highly original philosopher that he is most frequently read today. Is he less a scientist because he was originally inspired by a visit from "The Angel of Truth"? If modern cosmology is reviving alchemy, perhaps we should embrace more of the so-called myths of the foundations of our science. Terence and Dennis McKenna in their book, *The Invisible Landscape*, write that all science has origins in myth and they quote from Hans Jonas's essay on immortality.

What we commonly think of as science, whether it is nutrition, medicine, physics or chemistry, is still largely based on the concepts dating back as far as Isaac Newton, Plato and Aristotle. Medicinal and nutritional information still rely on studies of dead matter and tend to ignore the enzymatic processes of living matter. Often, we are limited to chemical formulas and physical equations that

9

are incapable of offering explanations for the processes of life. Einstein and others took us beyond the concept of molecules and atoms. We now know that atoms are subject to energetic influences from within our own bodies, from the magnetic fields of the earth, from solar energy and light, from the energy of what we ingest or apply to our bodies, and other energetic influences that can arrange and rearrange the components of the atoms that make up living matter. We still operate under disproved hypotheses and shallow concepts that stop at the structure of the atom.

Antoine Lavoisier introduced quantitative measurement into the study of chemistry with his discovery of the law of conservation of mass. He published the first chemistry text book in 1789. *Elements of Chemistry* is considered the foundation of chemistry. While his work led to the establishment of the periodic table, his belief that the atom was absolute would be overturned by the progress of scientific knowledge. However, Lavoisier's Law is still taught. Chemistry is a study of matter at the level of the atom or the molecules formed by atoms. Physics is a study of dead matter. Most chemists and physicists have closed their minds to anything that goes beyond the level of the atom because they see the human body with a convenient mechanics that can be explained by hypothetical equations.

The emerging microbiologists have found that the single cell life forms are capable of many transmutations and that they have intelligence for survival. Each cell of living matter has the same intelligence and ability to transmutate. We have believed for many years that atoms were the smallest forms of matter consisting of a nucleus and some protons. Today more than two hundred forms of subatomic particles have been identified, and we know that in living matter these particles can be rearranged to form different elements.

We are often too quick to embrace hypothesis as fact or truth. When we do we isolate ourselves from nature and close our minds to the wonderful mysteries of life. We suffer and toil. We spend years rowing our boat against the currents. We are so impressed with ourselves and our knowledge that we bring harm in the name of healing and destruction in the name of progress. We boast that we have conquered all the major infectious diseases when in the process we have created a host of environmental diseases. We are becoming victims of diseases that are not infectious. Heart disease, diabetes, osteoporosis, cancer and similar conditions are robbing us of the quality life science promised us. We are doing permanent damage to the earth and our bodies as we stray more and more from the natural path.

We produce more food than any other civilization in modern history, and we have more diet-related diseases than any other civilization in history. Actually, I recently learned of a civilization that existed in northern Peru that may have been the lost Atlantis and that may have had more productive farming methods than we have today. They used irrigation trenches and organic, sustainable methods to produce an abundance of food. Famine around the world does not come from an inability to produce food. Despite our green revolution of the past decades, famine is caused by corrupt and oppressive politics. Modern agriculture is based on the use of artificial fertilizers and other chemicals to control pests, weeds and growth. The primary component of our farming system is a form of nitrogen that is isolated from fossil fuel with extreme heat, also created from fossil fuel. Nitrogen is one of the most plentiful elements in our universe. In nature and organic or sustainable farming the nitrogen is released in the soil by microbes in a symbiotic

relationship with plants. Nitrogen is needed for growth. Our artificial fertilizer makes things grow, but at a great cost. Not only do we produce big beautiful fruits and vegetables with compromised nutritional value, but also the runoff is killing our waterways. Nitrogen means *without life*. The rivers have carried the runoff to the seas. In the Gulf of Mexico there is a "dead zone" larger than the state of New Jersey from the nitrogen carried by the Mississippi River. A few years ago a book was published that everybody should read. I put it in a category equal to *Silent Spring*. *Fatal Harvest* should be required reading in our country. It came on the literary scene with proper fanfare, but faded quickly. Perhaps its price, about double that of the average hardcover book, had something to do with its short lived interest. I could also believe that it is too depressing and filled with too many horrors for some people to handle. *Fatal Harvest* shows vividly the harm we are doing to our planet with the chemicals and farming practices we use to produce our food. We are doing similar harm to our bodies and the bodies of our children.

In 1624 Sir Francis Bacon with his *New Atlantis* put the "thinking" world on a journey to reclaim and conquer nature for the betterment of mankind. Science was God's way of leading us to the promised land. We may have been presumptuous, or greed may have clouded our concept of betterment. Whatever defines this journey, it has lost respect for mankind and the planet. Bacon saw nature as chaos that could be reclaimed and organized with science. Perhaps, the clear vision sees nature as having order and harmony and our "thinking" world as the source of chaos. Just because science could no longer fit the ancient mystical concepts of God into a progressive paradigm, it was easier to simply dismiss His existence. We have learned too much about our natural world to create a God in our own image, but we have not learned enough to comprehend the magnitude of Intelligence.

What does all this have to do with osteoporosis? **Everything.**

Later I will discuss the proven hypothesis of biological transmutation. It involves the ability of living matter to transmute one or more elements into another element. Scientists have accomplished transmutations of matter through nuclear fission and fusion. Experiments have succeeded in producing synthetic gold. These mutations however require extreme heat and other conditions that are very costly and impractical for everyday applications. Living matter on the other hand, has the ability to biologically transmute elements. Understanding the basics of biological transmutation opens the door to a deeper examination of nutrition and the use of dietary supplements.

Industrial scientists are on the verge of completely skipping quantum science as they prepare to move into the applications of nanno science. Quantum science goes beyond the atom to the point of interface with spiritual and energetic influences. Nanno science reverts to the molecular level and seals substances to retard aging. Nanno applications will give food products a longer shelf life, but reduce, or possibly lockout, the nutritional contents. Our food is already adulterated to the point of immorality. Nanno treatments may literally seal our fate to more diet related diseases.

In most cases osteoporosis is a diet related disease. As I

said earlier, there are hormonal and glandular problems that can cause bone loss as one of the symptoms. Most bone break and bone loss, however, come from deficiencies in the diet of the victim. Our Newtonian and Lavoisier approach to nutrition has led us to ingest calcium in ever increasing amounts to meet the needs of our bodies. This has not worked. Recent studies show that taking too much calcium from diet or supplements can actually contribute to bone break. A greater percentage of the people over fifty who experience bone breaks have good bone mass. Obviously there is more involved in bone health than mass or density. The quality of the bone must be a major factor in whether the person will suffer a fracture or not.

Our most modern concepts of osteoporosis are based on the relatively new methods of measuring bone mineral density, BMD.

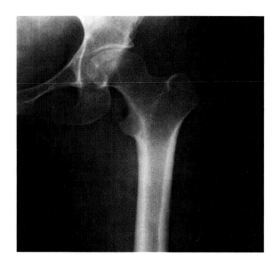

A BRIEF HISTORY OF
THE BONE DENSITY TESTS

The bone mineral density test, BMD, measures the density of bone matter and allows an estimation concerning the strength of the bones. The test involves the use of special x-ray, computed tomography (CTscan) or ultra sound. There are several procedures for conducting a BMD and the one chosen will most likely depend on cost and the amount of radiation exposure during the procedure.

DEXA, dual-energy x-ray absorptiometry, uses two x-ray beams. Bones with higher mineral density will block more of the x-beams. DEXA is the most often used test procedure and considered to be the most accurate. It also focuses on the hip and spine, the two areas most vulnerable to infirmity from excessive bone loss. The DEXA BMD can show as little as a 2% loss of bone from previous readings. DEXA is quick and easy with lower levels of radiation exposure. DEXA is more costly than other methods, however. SXA, single-energy x-ray absorptiometry is less expensive and also carries low levels of radiation exposure. However, SXA is limited to measurements of the bones of the forearm or heel.

P-DEXA, peripheral dual-energy x-ray absorptiometry, is a modification of DEXA. P-DEXA is not effective for measuring the BMD of the spine or hip, however. It is limited to measuring the limbs and does not show the areas where stress tends to cause the most fractures, the lower spine and the hip. DPA, dual photon absorptiometry, is low in radiation and it can measure the hip and spine. DPA has a much slower scan time and takes much longer that the other methods.

Ultrasound does not expose the patient to radiation and is the method most often used, initially. If an ultrasound examination of the heel indicates bone loss, the patient can be given a DEXA for confirmation. Ultrasound is convenient, but although it does not involve radiation, it is limited in its effectiveness because it does not measure BMD where fractures are more likely to occur, the spine and hip.

QCT, quantitative computed tomography, can be used to test BMD in the lower spine; however, it is expensive and has a higher exposure to radiation. QCT is also considered less accurate that DEXA. P-DEXA or DPA.

Development of the BMD test was a major break through in the diagnosis and treatment of osteoporosis. Before the BMD it was not possible to measure the amount of bone loss a patient was experiencing. Now a physician can know accurately the amount of bone a patient has lost.

The BMD is a powerful diagnostic tool when a person's readings are compared to a bell curve of readings from other patients of similar age and race living in the same climate. It is also very effective for comparison to a patient's own previous tests.

The BMD was introduced in the 90s by the World Health Organization with the enthusiastic support of a couple of pharmaceutical firms. Since the test was new, a standard was needed for comparisons. The standard was based on what the pharmaceuticals and the WHO assumed would be the peak or ideal bone mass for a 30 year old Caucasian woman in perfect health. Two standards were set, "young normal" and "age-matched". Young normal is known as the T-score and the BMD is used to estimate the possibility of bone fracture against the assumed ideal or peak mass of the nonexistent 30 year old healthy woman. Age-matched readings are called the Z-score, and again are based on assumptions of what would be ideal for a person of similar age. Lower BMD scores are common among older women, and even the estimated norm for the age-matched comparisons can be very misleading to say the least.

A T-score within one marker or standard deviation (SD) of the bone mass of the ideal thirty year old is considered normal. 1-2.5 SDs below the arbitrary norm is diagnosed as osteopinia. Many observers have concluded that osteopenia is more a marketing term that a medical condition. A Z-score of more than 2.5 SDs is diagnosed as osteoporosis. Suddenly, hundreds of thousands of women were eligible for the new bisphosphonate type drugs.

The body builds bone mass via osteoblasts, a combination of nutrients that converts to healthy bone mass. The body gives up bone mass via osteoclasts. In a healthy body the skeleton is constantly giving off osteoclasts and replacing them with fresh osteoblasts. Presumably, even in older people with reduced bone mass, a balance between osteoblasts and osteoclasts can be maintained. The body uses the osteoclasts from the skeleton to control the pH and to maintain balance among various minerals. The surrender of bone mass to control these balances is a very important process. For example, if the pH becomes too acid, oxygen is reduced and bacteria or cancer cells can thrive in the carbon rich environment.

The bisphosphonate drugs block the creation of osteoclasts thereby preserving bone mass. These drugs do little to build new bone, other than block the erosion of bone mass. They do not directly enhance the production of osteoblasts, although vitamin D has been added to some of them. Within weeks of starting these antiresorptive drugs the body actually decreases the formation of new bone. As a result the remaining bone is less prone to fracture, but it is not youthful or healthy bone mass. While bisphosphonate drugs may be helpful to a person in crisis, the long term use of them is coming under increased questioning. Several class action lawsuits have been started against some of the makers of these drugs because of the side effects. One condition linked to a bisphosphonate is osteonecrosis of the jaw or "dead jaw' according to an article in the professional publication, *Journal of Oral and Maxillofacial Surgeons.*

On countless occasions young women in their late thirties and early forties came to my store in distress, often depressed. They had just been told that they had osteopenia and were given a prescription for a bisphosphonate drug. I would explain how the drug worked and encourage them to also concentrate on supplements and a diet that would provide the nutrients needed to promote healthy bone mass by creating new bone.

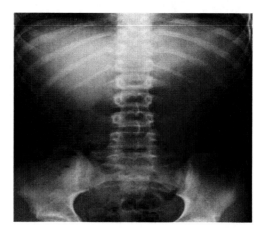

MY PERSONAL EVOLUTION

"Lavoisier was a great scholar of the 18th century. He is considered the father of modern chemistry. The general principle with which he worked and from which he derived his new science is that nothing is lost, nothing is created, everything is transformed. The atom being considered the smallest particle of matter and a constant in nature, it was assumed that no element could be created. This principle could in way be refuted or even debated. It was not until the 20th century that this principle, left undiscussed for more than one hundred years saw its first officially recognized contradiction."

Louis Kervran

.

By sharing my personal evolution and convictions concerning supplementing for bone health, I can also give you a review of current thinking in the industry and among health care professionals who have a nutritional orientation. In the mid 90s when I decided the best venue to sell my herbs would be in a health food store, I began an intensive study program on nutrition and the use of supplements and herbs. At the time, I was in the common Lavoisier mode, believing that people who consumed milk and dairy products were getting good calcium. The Lavoisier mindset emphasized calcium for bone health, and dairy contains calcium. So I naturally believed that dairy or soy and other products fortified with calcium were desirable. All of the available literature suggested that women should supplement their diets with 1000 to 1200 mg of calcium daily and consume several servings of dairy or other calcium fortified food.

As I progressed, it became clear that vitamin D was of major importance for building and maintaining healthy bone mass. Years earlier it was discovered that children with rickets, a bone disorder, needed vitamin D. Milk comes fortified with vitamin D; unfortunately, it is fortified with synthetic forms for the vitamin, D1 or D2. The true sunshine vitamin is D3. Vitamin D3 is the form made by the body in sunlight and the form that is needed for bone health. Actually vitamin D3 is a hormone more than a vitamin, and its value to the human body goes far beyond healthy bones. It is one of the most important nutrients supporting the immune system against several forms of cancer. In the last decade as more was learned about vitamin D3 the recommended daily allowance has grown from a 200 iu to at least 400 iu. Based on the latest studies manyexprts now suggest 2000 iu or more for some people. The need is usually based on the amount of sunlight the person experiences daily. Climate is also a factor in determining the amount of vitamin D a person should consume daily as a supplement. People living near the equator where sunshine in plentiful every day need less supplemental vitamin D than people living in the colder zones of the earth. Their need also varies between winter and summer. At my store we offered an excellent vitamin D. Most vitamin D supplements come from fish oils such as cod liver oil. These forms also contain oil soluble vitamin A on a ratio of 10 to 1. The one we offered, and is still offered at Pleasant Stone Farm comes from lamb's wool and contains no vitamin A. Customers could take 1000 iu or more without concerns of overloading on vitamin A.

As more studies became available, it became clear that magnesium was important for bone health. Most of the preferred supplements would contain vitamin D3 and magnesium. Usually the magnesium would be at a level of half in relation to the calcium. Many were suggesting that the supplement contain equal parts of calcium and magnesium.

I did intensive studies for more than a year prior to opening the store. Pleasant Stone Farm opened in a strip mall on Dolson Ave in Middletown, NY on April 1, 1997. I was reading good studies from reliable journals, but when I started working face to face with my customers, the education and learning process really began. First hand information from people with a personal experience with an herb or supplement was superior to reading about studies in even the most prestigious journals. Soon, I was hearing complaints from people, mostly women, who were experiencing difficult side effects from the high levels of calcium they were taking. I remember one woman whose doctor had told her to take 2000 mg of calcium daily suffered extreme constipation.

As more information became available it was clear that the kind of calcium was very important. Several studies showed that while calcium carbonate might be good for heartburn (as in Tums) it did not absorb well. In fact, the calcium carbonate formed a sludge-like substance when it encountered stomach acid. It was good for neutralizing the acid and relieving heartburn, but it was constipating and not likely to reach the bones. Calcium citrate was being touted as the better form of calcium. Many doctors are still telling their patients to take Tums for their calcium. I believe this is a perfect example of the inadequacy of the Lavoisier mindset for determining our nutritional needs.

With these developments my own personal conflicts with calcium began to take shape. The human bone contains calcium carbonate. Why would calcium carbonate not be the best form to supplement a diet or fortify a food? It would be a couple of years before I would get the answer. I came across many studies that concluded people experienced no improvement in bone mass after years of taking calcium supplements. One of the largest long term studies ever undertaken, concluded that women taking 1000 mg of calcium did not show any change in bone mass. This was the third part of the massive, million-woman study that was called to a halt because it found that estrogen and progesterone actually increased heart disease and some forms of cancer. The impact of the study on HRT got all the attention and the calcium supplementation was seldom mentioned. Usually I dismissed the reports on the uselessness of calcium supplementation when they were based on the use of calcium carbonate. When calcium citrate or other forms of the mineral were used, and there was little or no improvement in bone mass, the confusion mounted. During this period I remember a study of geriatric patients who failed to show improvement from supplementing calcium citrate. It was the confusion that kept me searching for more solid information on supplementing for bone mass.

I began to suggest that customers try MCHA, microcrystalline calcium hydroxyapatite. MCHA is made from calf bone. It has the same ratio of components as human bone. In addition to calcium and magnesium, MCHA contains potassium, zinc, phosphorous and other support minerals. For the first time I was suggesting a calcium supplement with some confidence. I arranged to offer it under the Pleasant Stone Farm label. We sourced it out of New Zealand. New Zealand does not have the acid rain, dioxin and other pollutants in its ecosystem that we have in the United States. Within a few months customers were thanking me, because their bone mineral density test showed they were adding bone mass. Again, it is important to study reports on good scientific studies, but nothing is better than the personal experience of a person who has used a product, successfully. This is why I believe that my customers have taught me more than all the books and journals I have read.

I came to believe that the MCHA from calf bone absorbed better than the other forms of calcium supplements because it was a food form that would digest and assimilate. I was able to improve on MCHA with a product we called Bone Strength, by adding vitamin K, Boron and Horsetail. Vitamin K is essential for the production of the osteoblasts the body uses to replace bone mass. Boron is essential for healthy joints and connective tissue. Horsetail is rich in silica which the body uses to make healthy bones. Silica also helps produce collagen which enhances hair, skin and nails.

As I became more aware of the antiquated thinking and concepts of nutrition based on Lavoisier's chemistry, I began to doubt the value of calcium as a supplement or food additive. Finally I was led to discover online a little, out of print book by a French scientist, Louis Kervran, on biological transmutation. The Lavoisier mindset thinks that calcium is always calcium, magnesium is always magnesium and that all of the elements are absolute. This mindset taught us that the atom is the smallest particle of an element. Plank and Einstein however, showed us that the atom can be split. They showed us that the atom is made of energetic particles. Change the number of protons or neutrons with energetic particles from other elements and the makeup of the atom changed, or transmuted, into another element.

Scientists have been able to make diamonds and gold by subjecting elements to extreme heat. The process of using heat to release nitrogen changed agriculture, and it provided us with limitless explosives to harm our neighbors, or be harmed by them. Kervran documented the biological transmutation of elements and assembled the findings of other scientists.

Kervran devotes most of his writing to the transmutation of elements in the sprouting of seeds. The sprouts will contain elements not found in the seed. In other words, living matter can enzymatically change the structure of atoms without high heat or extreme laboratory conditions.

He writes that as a child on his grandparents farm, he watched the chickens scratch and consume small particles of mica. Later when he would open the gizzard he would find grit, but no particles of mica. The chicken had transmuted the mica, a solid form of silica, into bone mass and other body parts. Later as a scientist he would show that the egg contained no calcium other than the shell, yet when the chick hatched, it would have a complete skeleton. Still on the farm Kervran notes that cows produce gallons and gallons of milk rich in calcium. They do so without suffering osteoporosis or bone loss. Cows given calcium supplements do not have an increased amount of calcium in their milk. The cow depends on magnesium and other minerals in good green pasture grass. The grass depends on calcium in the soil to produce grass that is rich in magnesium. In other words, the plants need calcium. Mammals need magnesium. Vegetation transmutes calcium into magnesium and mammals transmute magnesium into calcium to form healthy bones.

I now believe that it was not the calcium in the MCHA

That increased the bone mass of my customers. I believe it was the other minerals in the matrix that supplied them with the nutrients they needed to make bone mass. I now have come full cycle in my thinking. I agree with Dr Andrew Weil and others who have concluded that we should avoid calcium supplements. The cutting edge consensus today suggests actually that too much calcium can lead to unhealthy bone mass. This would explain why often people with the greater bone mass can suffer more broken bones. Their bones tend to crumble as it were. Excessive amounts of calcium could also deplete the skeleton of other vital minerals. For example, the brittle bone is magnesium and the flexibility and strength comes from the cords of calcium that surround it. Perhaps, too much calcium from excessive dairy consumption or supplementation can cause a deficit of magnesium as the body works to keep a proper ratio among minerals. We have learned much in the last decade; unfortunately, we are decades behind what we should have learned from Einstein and Planck nearly half a century ago. My only consolation is that while I may have completely reversed my thinking on the use of calcium supplements, my convictions always, have been on the cutting edge of emerging information.

I was working on the outline for this book in the spring of 2006. It was interrupted by a series of events that changed the course of our lives and redirected the journey. First, Lillian caught her heel in a metal strip getting out of a booth in a restaurant in Canton, Georgia. The fall broke her hip. She had good surgery at the local hospital in Canton, but when she was moved to a facility in Atlanta for her rehabilitation she was injured again. An aide helping her get into bed lifted the leg above her head and dislodged the prosthesis. She had to have a second much more complicated operation. By the time I got her home and barely on her feet, I came down with cancer. It was treated successfully and removed in February of 2007 in a ten hour procedure. I was too weak to work on the book until after the surgery. By the fall of 2007 I was working on it a little several times per week. Now in August of 2008 it is ready for the printer. I feel blessed in many ways, including having had more time to research and study.

When we embrace biological transmutation, we begin to get a completely different concept of agriculture and nutrition. We begin to understand more deeply the teachings of Einstein when he said that matter is energy and beyond that "supreme intelligence". When we go beyond the atom to its component parts we find the energy. Food becomes energy that enhances the energy of our body. It is a challenging frontier when we crack the shell of the atom. It is just as deep and fathomless as space. Perhaps in exploring the atom we will be able to bring ourselves closer to comprehending the Supreme Intelligence that energizes it.

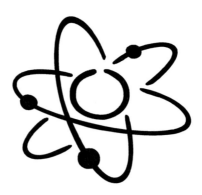

WHY DO SO MANY WOMEN HAVE
OSTEOPOROSIS TODAY?

Bones found during the restoration of a London church from people who were buried between 1729 and 1852 were examined for bone loss. It was concluded that modern women suffer more bone loss than women from earlier centuries. Bones of women in less developed parts of the world where their diets remain close to the earth, mostly devoid of modern conveniences, also show less bone loss than the modern woman. One is forced to believe that the modern diet is the cause of the epidemic of osteoporosis.

Osteoporosis, like heart disease, diabetes and most forms of cancer and arthritis are conditions that can be traced to diet. What we consume, or fail to consume, is killing more of us than the pandemics of history. We have been able to achieve at least limited or temporary control of infections, but we have created a mass metabolic-meltdown from the contamination and adulteration of our food. We have come to depend on thousands of chemicals more than the simple, natural and organic laws of horticulture. We are less interested in understanding nature and the mysteries of the embryo and more content with scientific tricks that empower our commercial goals. We can boast of many achievements, but they are costing us our health. Worse, we have sold the health of our children and enslaved ourselves to unachievable fantasies of convenience.

While we have learned to grow bigger and more abundant crops, we have neglected the basic purpose of food, nutrition. Thousands of years before Christ farmers were cultivating crops and saving seeds. As we read the ancient accounts of agriculture, we do not find many, or any, references to improved nutritional content. The focus has always been on production. There are many considerations: days to maturity, ability to withstand draught, ability to resist fungus, and shelf life after harvest. These are all important concerns for the farmers and merchants. Where is the concern for the consumer and the nutrition that is expected from the food? In ancient times nutrition was taken for granted; today nutrition has even less consideration.

About 250,000 plant species have been recorded. Of these, only some 200 are cultivated for food. Most of the food on our planet comes from as few as twenty crops in only eight food groups. Our food choices have been reduced dramatically in the last century. In the early 1900s American farmers were producing more than 500 varieties of cabbage. Today, fewer than thirty varieties of cabbage are cultivated. Similar reductions can be found in carrots, cauliflower, and many other fruits and vegetables. The fruits, vegetables and nuts in production today were all developed during ancient times by seed saving farmers.

The practice of saving seeds began to diminish in the 1940s with the discovery of "hybrid vigor". It was learned that seeds, cross pollinated with cousins or grandparent seeds would produce a bigger harvest.

Farmers began to depend on new seeds each planting season. The extra cost was justified by the higher yields. Soon a small handful of seed companies were controlling agriculture, not only in the United States, but also in other countries with mechanized farming. As the seed sources became narrower, the varieties within the species also were reduced. With the development of new hybrids each year and greater dependence on machinery, farmers were forced to depend more and more on chemical fertilizers, herbicides and pesticides.

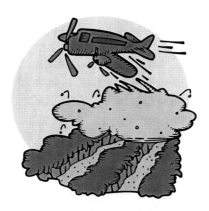

"We are still eating the leftovers from WWII"
Indian activist farmer,   Vandana Shiva

Some of these highly toxic chemicals are still pervasive in our environment and in our bodies years after they were banned. Hundreds more toxic chemicals are introduced each year with very little, if any, testing for their effect on humans and other animals or plants. The testing is left to the industry and negative findings are usually withheld from regulators. Only after harm is done, do these products get serious scrutiny. Most of the chemicals used to control pests and weeds originally, were made from stockpiles of WWII chemical weapons. These chemicals were too toxic to dump or store, so they were diluted and made into household and agricultural products.

As the varieties of food crops diminished agricultural officials in countries everywhere began to see the importance of saving heirloom seeds. More countries maintain seeds banks today than ever before and there are efforts to establish more than one international seed bank. When the courts allowed seeds to be treated as intellectual property and patents were issued, it became more difficult to save and exchange seeds. Suddenly farmers who had saved and cultivated seeds for centuries were forced to buy seeds. We average citizens have not been aware to the "seed wars" that have been raging globally for several years. Today, the situation is totally complicated by genetic tampering. GMOs, genetically modified organisms represent a larger percentage of farm acreage each year. In the United States an estimated 90% of the soy crops are GMOs. More and more GMOs are reaching the market in the United States, and there are no laws to restrict them despite extensive evidence that they might be harmful. Today control of agriculture is shifting from the seed companies to the chemical and pharmaceutical giants that are engaged in developing GMOs.

Personally, I believe that genetic modification is immoral. When hybrids are developed the process involves cross pollination between compatible plants. Genetic modification involves the introduction of genes from any life form into a plant or animal. Genes from fish, bacteria and various animals, including humans, have been spliced into plants. I believe this violates nature in a dangerous way and for that reason that is immoral. Many credible scientists are warning of the possibility of super weeds or other catastrophic developments from GMOs. Genetically modified fish are being raised in fish farms for human consumption. Many scientists believe if any of these modified species should escape and breed with wild fish, the entire population could be eliminated in three or four generations. Cloning and gene splicing are becoming an integral part of animal husbandry.

A poorly kept secret program involves splicing human genes into swine to develop a future harvest of organs for human transplant. Many plants have been genetically modified to produce pharmaceutical drugs, and there is a proven danger of these crops cross pollinating with food crops. There are links and suggested reading material on this subject in the resource section at the end of this book. By the way, yields from these "Franken-crops" have not met expectations and the only reports of success come from the companies that sell the seeds and the chemicals to support them, not from the farmers who are forced to use them.

Genetically modified strains of corn have contaminated the corn fields in the mountains of Mexico. There are documented cases of allergic reactions to GMO corn that was accidentally mixed with food products. GMO corn is approved for livestock feed. In the end what difference does it make. If I am what I eat, then so is the cow or other animal the sum of what it eats. So, if I eat the animal, I ultimately am consuming the GMOs. The purpose of genetic modification does not involve nutrition. Shelf life and chemicals are the focus. GMOs are developed to withstand herbicides, but they require more chemical pesticides. The corporations that make the GMOs naturally are the corporations that sell the chemicals. For the consumer this means more chemical residue and less nutrition.

If food is processed there is a high probability that it will contain one or more GMO ingredients. The four major GMO crops are corn, soy, cotton seed and canola. I have long marveled at the belief that canola oil is a health food. It comes from rape Seed. The rape seed was chosen because it will grow in the frigid Canadian climates. Rape seed is toxic and was not a successful cattle feed. After it was genetically modified to remove its toxins, the cattle still rejected it. The oil from the genetically modified rape seed became Canadian Oil, Canola for short. It has somehow found its way into the health market as a good oil. I do not share that opinion. Read the labels. You will find corn, soy, canola and cotton seed in almost every food that is factory processed. The food processors are careful to keep the GMOs out of food that is produced for the European markets because consumers have rejected them. In the US most consumers are not aware of the GMOs and there are no label requirements. However, if one wants to know if a fruit or vegetable is a GMO, simply look at the numbers of the item. If it starts with an 8, it is an organic product. If it starts with a 9 it is genetically modified. If it starts with 1 to 7, it is a conventional product. With the 2008 crop year many more GMOs will be grown in the US including sugar beets.

There are a few biotech companies alleging to address nutrition with new GMO products. There is an effort to develop so-called yellow or golden rice. The idea is to genetically modify the rice to make it contain more vitamin A. If it is successful, it will contain lesser amounts of other nutrients. Another commercial folly involves genetically modifying carrots to contain more calcium. I can just imagine Bugs Bunny becoming a spokesman for "calcicarrots". Our health problems will never be addressed successfully by greed and adulteration of life forms. The cradle of agriculture is Iraq. Records show that Iraqi farmers were cultivating crops 6,750 years before Christ. There are earlier records from Mesopotamia dating to 8000 BC. Ancient seeds from Mesopotamia were stored in Iraq's seed bank in the town of Abu Ghraib. Heirloom varieties of chick peas, lentils and grains were housed there. In March, 2003 during the US invasion, the seed bank was looted and destroyed.

Some seeds were saved because alert officials had placed some of the seeds in a simple cardboard box and sent them to Syria. When these seeds are returned to a new seed bank in Iraq some day, Iraqi farmers may not have access to them. Currently, Iraqi farmers have to buy seeds from Monsanto or Dow Chemical, the two leading giants in developing GMOs. Iraqi farmers have been restricted from saving seeds because of international patents. When they use the GMOs their remaining heirlooms will surely be contaminated by them.

I often think it might be easier to sell our "American style democracy" if freedom did not come with corporate strings attached. We Americans take our corruptions in stride. They are insulated under many layers of pseudo patriotism and adulterated history. Perhaps we have to realize that an Iraqi farmer experiencing the sensitive nerve ends of current events may find it difficult to believe that buying seeds from Dow or Monsanto is a newly gained freedom. They might also want to know why they have to pay a premium for a patent on a seed cultivated on their land by their great grandfathers.

In Afghanistan, during the 2001 overthrow of the Taliban scientists removed seeds from the bank in Kabul and hid them in jars in two houses in Ghazni and Jalalabad. Fruits and nuts developed in the region were involved. Grapes, melons, cherries, plums, peaches, apricots, pears and rare varieties of almonds and walnuts were being protected in the Afghan bank. When they returned to the houses both had been looted. The seeds were found dumped on the floor. Apparently, the thieves only found the jars to be of value; they left the seeds. Afghan farmers may not realize the loss in the near future. Most are engaged in the cultivation of poppies for the world drug trade.

Sadly, agriculture is entangled in world politics. The small farmer is suffering. The consumers are suffering. The lack of nutrition from the food available to us, is causing diseases. The root cause of osteoporosis, heart disease, diabetes, arthritis, cancer and other food related diseases is politics and the greed that drives it. The greed and corruption begin with the seeds, but corruption can be found at every level and in every step between the field and the table. In the United States in the name of price stabilization, billions of dollars are shifted from tax payers to well connected farm interests each year. The Farm Bill underwrites junk food. The junk food appears to be a bargain because side by side with organic or more nutritious food in the market, it has a lower price. Most Americans believe that nutritious food is too expensive. What they do not realize is that the junk food that appears to be a bargain comes with hidden subsides from their own pocket. When we realize that it is the chemically toxic junk food underwritten by our tax money that is the cause of our mass metabolic meltdown, we should realize that we are supporting the primary cause of our run-away health care costs.

Time Magazine, June 23, 2008 reported in a series of articles on childhood obesity that the cost of fresh fruits and vegetables rose between 1989 and 2005 by 74.6%. During that same period *Time* reports there was a reduction in the cost of junk and fat foods of 26.5%. If we want to do something to stop the rising cost of health care, we could begin by stopping the tax supported farm bill that perpetuates our junk food eating habits. The issue is not that organic and nutritious food costs more. The true issue is how much we could save in political give-aways and health care by making better food choices. We would also see savings in education, crime and correction, and worker productivity. Also, if the government stopped supporting the factory-farm concept of agriculture, we would see a surge in community, sustainable farming with a leveling of prices and an abundance of fresh, healthy food.

According to *Food Review* hip fractures are the most serious consequence of osteoporosis. About 20 percent result in death, and those who survive often have disability and loss of independence. Osteoporosis-related hip fractures result in estimated costs of $12.8 billion to $17.8 billion per year for medical care, extended treatment facilities, and the value of lost productivity. Rehabilitation and institutionalization costs, at about $5.1 billion to $7.1 billion, account for 40 percent of the estimated total economic cost of osteoporosis-related hip fractures. The value of lost productivity due to missed work is less than 1 percent of total economic costs, while value of premature death accounts for 35.3 percent. Initial medical costs for hospitalization and outpatient care, at about $3.1 billion to $4.3 billion, account for 24.4 percent of the total economic cost of osteoporosis-related hip fractures. By the way, these figures come from research done ten years ago. The costs are much higher today. If we consumed more quality food, we would have a better quality of life and save billions of dollars.

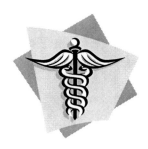

NITROGEN, MAKES THINGS GROW

AND KILLS THE EARTH

In 1841 John Bennet Lawes built the world's first fertilizer factory and began selling "superphosphate", and agriculture would never be the same. Lawes actually took the discoveries of Justus von Liebig who is historically the "father of the fertilizer industry". Lawes however took out patents while Justus von Liebig was publishing scientific papers. Little wonder that today piracy and patents are at the core of mechanized agriculture. That was its beginning.

German scientist Fritz Haber was awarded the Nobel prize in 1918 for "improving the standards of agriculture and the well being of mankind". Haber several years earlier had developed a way to isolate nitrogen atoms. Haber, however, was more interested in using nitrogen for explosives in support of the German war effort in WWI. Haber developed poison gas, chlorine and ammonia. He also developed Zyklon b, the gas used by Hitler's forces for concentration camp exterminations. Nitrogen is the explosive agent in the fertilizer used in making bombs such as the one that destroyed the Federal Building in Oklahoma City. Fertilizer was also used in the first attack on the World Trade Center.

Each year agriculture becomes more dependent on fossil

fuels for production and delivery. Food raised with modern methods and from genetically modified seeds require more chemical support than older conventional or organic crops. The chemicals involved in agriculture are made from coal tar and crude oil. In addition, the average food item on the grocery shelf has traveled 1,500 miles. Aside from the added expense for fuel, the long distance the food will travel is time consuming. For this reason, most crops are harvested green or immature. In the life cycle of a plant or fruit, most of the time on the vine is spent growing to a full size. Once the item reaches full size, it begins to make vitamins and antioxidants from photosynthesis in the sun as the roots begin to take in minerals from the earth. If the harvest takes place before the product is ripe, there is less opportunity for it to acquire the desired nutrients. Harvesting before a crop is fully mature or ripe reduces the nutrition. If a peach has to travel 1,500 miles to market, there is no mystery as to why it is hard as a rock or rots before it ripens. We must depend more on regional agriculture and sustainable farming methods if we are to reverse the illnesses that are so prevalent today.

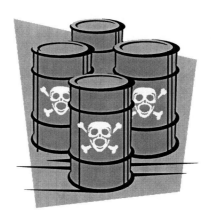

TO CONSRVE OIL WE ARE BURNING FOOD

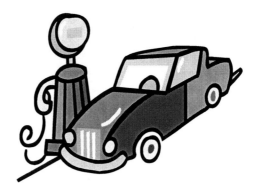

The cost of crude oil is causing food prices to rise, not only for the transportation of food items over the average 1,500 miles, but also for the production of the chemicals needed to support modern style factory farms. Personally, I think this situation is going to be made more severe for the American food budget. The price of a basic commodity, corn, is rising steadily despite record setting abundant harvests, and it is not because we are eating more corn or feeding more of it to livestock. We are converting corn to ethanol to reduce our dependence on oil imports. The price of wheat and other grains is rising and food riots broke out around the world in early 2008. Flour for bread rose drastically in price as farmers switched from wheat to corn and other crops for the biofuel market. Biofuel from corn sounds like a good idea, until we realize that it takes more oil to produce the corn than the ethanol can replace. Yes, it takes more oil to produce and process the corn into ethanol. Aside from the fact that ethanol from corn is financially counter productive, we are burning food.

Originally, the diesel engine was invented to run on corn or other vegetable oils. When it threatened the status quo of the powerful oil interests, fuel oil was made available at gas stations for the diesel powered vehicles. This put transportation with the diesel engine in competition with the furnaces used for heating homes. We not only transport food an average 1,500 miles, we transport nearly all of our goods via diesel-powered trucks. When diesel replaced vegetable oils as engine fuel, the next step was the creation of the edible oil industry. Corn and other vegetable oils with the help of slick public relations replaced healthy saturated fats. America began cooking with vegetable shortening and spreading margarine on toast. Heart disease and other conditions began to rise dramatically. I will talk more about what I call "junk oils" shortly. If you want to know more about the relationship between the grain lobby and the agencies that set policy for our food, you might like to read my book, *The Amber Waves of Gain, How the Government Makes Us Fat.*

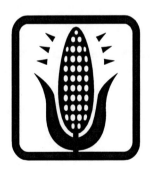

DOES YOUR FOOD COME FROM THE EARTH

OR A FACTORY?

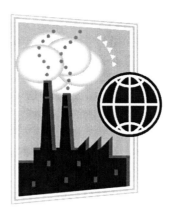

Each year a greater percentage of our food is processed. Even fresh fruits and vegetables are subjected to processing before reaching the supermarket shelves. Irradiation has become a common practice in preparing food for market. The industry likes to refer to this process as "electronic pasteurization". Fruits, vegetables and meat products are placed in vaults with concrete walls that are three feet thick. The thick walls protect workers from the radiation. Industry officials and officials at the regulatory agencies claim the food is not harmed by the radiation, that it only kills fungus and bacteria. Studies show that the radiation is equal to 350,000 chest x-rays and that it does change the molecular structure of the foods. Most agree it is enough to damage the amino acids, vitamins and antioxidants reducing the nutritional value of the food. The government refuses to require labeling of food that is irradiated, which of course is consistent with the history of our regulatory agencies. After 9/11 and the anthrax scare in Washington, mail sent to government officials and members of Congress was irradiated to kill anthrax or other germs that might have been planted by terrorists. These government officials, who have refused to be concerned with the safety of our food after irradiation, suddenly were concerned about touching their mail after it was "electronically pasteurized". I found this too to be historically consistent with the attitude toward the citizens and tax payers.

Distribution centers have special houses or storage facilities for such products as bananas and tomatoes where they can be treated with chemicals and gasses to make them appear to be ripe. Both are picked green and treated hours before being put on the shelves for purchase. So you see, even "fresh" produce is processed and treated. It is common now for supermarkets and food processors to treat red meat with carbon monoxide to prolong the red or fresh color.

More and more the food reaching the American tables comes from a factory. At one of the local supermarkets my wife and I use, we noticed that the frozen section has been devoted almost completely to processed or factory based foods. The selection of vegetables has been reduced to include only the store brand in about four doors of one freezer section. The remainder including one large isle of coffin-type freezers offers every conceivable cut of French fry, infinite choices of waffles, and complete meals. We Americans have the biggest and best equipped kitchens in history. At no time have the masses had the refrigeration, stoves, and gadgets that are common in the

41

kitchen of the average American home today. At no time have Americans consumed more food from restaurants and food processors than today. Cookbooks sales have never been higher. We have complete cable channels devoted to cooking. There are numerous magazines dedicated to the preparation of food. One would assume that we are all cooking more. Truth is, we are using these wonderful kitchens to thaw and heat processed food. Very little time is spent actually *cooking*.

Factory processing involves more chemical additives. First, the food comes from the fields chemical laden. Then the processor will use more chemicals to enhance the flavor and appearance, and still more chemicals to preserve it. Every step of processing reduces nutritional content and every step involves one or more additional chemicals. These chemicals are known to be toxic, but their use is approved at very low levels. However, there is no consideration of the cumulative effect of exposure to them over time. Neither is there consideration of the increased toxicity when these chemicals are combined with others. Despite the millions of tax dollars we give to the governments to protect us, the agencies that regulate our food remain cozy with the industry. The success of these agencies of government is measured by financial statistics and gross sales. In other words, the regulatory agencies have an agenda that will insure growth of the industry. The safety of the consumer and the nutritional needs of the nation are lost in the greed and corruption that drive the political system. Consequently, we are denied access to nutritious food and brain-washed to believe that what is put before us is safe and wholesome. We are also led to believe that our national problem with weight and obesity comes from our lack of exercise. Actually, our obesity comes primarily from a handful of sources, and their impact on our health is obvious. Refined grains, high fructose corn syrup, processed vegetable oils and chemical additives such as MSG are among the primary causes of our obesity and metabolic health crisis.

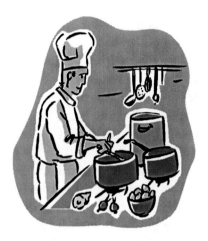

If food is prepared in a commercial kitchen or factory processed it will be reduced in nutritional value and most likely contain more than one toxic substance to enhance flavor, appearance and shelf life.

THE WHITES

I am sure by this time in the movement toward more organic eating that you have heard about the "whites". In the production of white rice and white flour, the most nutritious parts of the kernel are removed leaving only the starchy part that nature put into the seed to feed the sprouting embryo. Wheat, barley, rye, oats, rice and other grains are plants from the grass family and the grains are their seeds. We remove the fiber, bran and kernel in processing them into modern flour. The move is toward a resumption of whole grain foods. Whole grain simply means that the best part of the seed has not been removed. White flour makes a fluffy cake and a flaky biscuit, but it also makes fat and contributes to obesity. Rice bran is loaded with all kinds of nutrients, some of which are classified as miracle foods when they are isolated. Wheat and other grains, like all their grassy cousins, need calcium to grow and produce magnesium. In the processing the magnesium is lost. This is why eating processed foods such as the whites can contribute to the diseases that are rampant among us today. We need the magnesium to avoid osteoporosis. We fortify and supplement with tons of calcium, but we must realize that calcium is not doing the job or replacing the nutrition processing has removed.

The whites are: white flour, white rice, refined sugar, refined salt and milk. Nutrition gives food a color. Making them white removes the nutrition. Just think for a minute about the percentage of a daily diet that is made up of the "whites" and it becomes clear why people on the check out line in the supermarket and their families look like what they have put into their carts.

THE FINAL MUTILATION

The mutilation of our food does not end with the factory processing, it continues in our designer kitchens with the microwave. Why would we want to put our food into a contraption that kills everything. The microwave has become central to American cuisine. We even have experts telling us that microwaving vegetables in a phthalate-laden plastic bag delivers more nutrition than boiling or steaming. I am compelled to include a brief history of the microwave.

The microwave was developed by German scientists. They were looking for ways to feed their army as it marched to Warsaw. The microwave cooked without fuel. The German army was thwarted from invading Russia, and in the spoils of war Russia gained possession of the microwave technology. After a few years of study the Russians abandoned the device because of its undesirable effects on food. In the early 90s scientists in Switzerland proved that the microwave created radiotrons and changed the molecular structure of items that were subjected to its radiation. A radiotron is described as a substance that never existed before. In other words, the microwave changes ordinary food into an alien substance.

The information was suppressed and plans to put a microwave in every home and office in the United States proceeded. The microwave mutilates vital enzymes, vitamins, amino acids and other nutrients in the food cooked or warmed in it. Does this contribute to osteoporosis and other diet related diseases?

WE CHOOSE GOOD OIL FOR OUR CARS,

AND JUNK OIL FOR OUR BODIES

Junk oil in the diet is a major cause of obesity as our bodies store fats that cannot be metabolized. Trans fats have finally been exposed, but the effort to get rid of them has been vastly ridiculed. I cringe when I see and hear a news reporter make some ignorant comment after covering a story concerning a food item like trans fats. The industry came up with a spin on trans fats that is comparable only to the public relations people who spoke out for the safety of cigarettes years ago. The industry would have us believe that the only trans fats are the vegetable oils that have been partially hydrogenated. Many vegetable or seed oils become tans fats when they are heated above 220 degrees Fahrenheit, and most of them are heated that much and more several times during their preparation for market. Trans fats are an inorganic substance in the body. This is the fat that clogs the arteries, surrounds the organs and flabs our least curvaceous body parts.

Two of these oils are pervasive in our diets, even if we think we are avoiding them. Corn and soy oils are products that are refined for use in food in many chemical forms. Read the labels; you have no idea how often you are consuming these two products. In one form or another they are in everything with the blessings of the regulator agencies. Corn and soy are the foundation of American agriculture. Not only do we consume them in some form in hundreds of processed foods, we also consume them second hand in all the animal products that reach our table.

We know now that saturated fats were sacrificed on the alter of commerce when the edible oil industry was being created. Ironically when McDonalds made French fries in lard and tallow, they were less harmful than those made in the hydrogenated oil they used to replace the saturated fats. Bowing to public pressure again, they have switched from the tans fat to soy oil. According to Udo Erasmus who wrote *Fats That Heal, Fats That Kill,* vegetable oils heated above 220 degrees Fahrenheit take on the trans fat characteristics. The heat changes the structure of the molecule from a rod to a bent rod. Most vegetable and seed oils are heated above 220 degrees several times during the processing that prepares them for market.

Vegetable and seed oils can have many desirable qualities when they are first rendered, but they quickly oxidize or go rancid. By the time they reach the bottling plant they are rancid and cloudy. Many times hexane, or gasoline, is used to remove the last drops of oil from the pulp. One heating process is the distillation that removes the hexane from the oil. The cloudiness is removed with degreasers similar to those used in window cleaners and drain openers. Finally, we have a beautifully clear oil, but it still stinks from having gone rancid. The final process is boiling to remove the odor and rancid taste. When the processing is done it is hard to tell one vegetable or seed oil from another. It is sold as vegetable oil, or made into vegetable shortening.

We have been told by the health community that these highly processed oils are better for us. We replaced butter with margarine and lard with shortening. The truth is, while an abundance of saturated fat in the diet can be a challenge, even a small amount of trans fat is a challenge. Our bodies convert saturated fat to energy. We convert trans fat to body fat.

IF IT AINT BROKE DON'T FIX IT

IF IT AINT SICK TREAT IT ANYHOW

Years ago farmers found that feeding soy to animals acted on the thyroid gland and slowed metabolism. Animals consuming soy gained more weight. They also found that adding corn to the feed increased weight gain. They quickly learned that the corn oil reduced immune levels of the animals. So the drugs they had given the animals to slow their metabolism were replaced by antibiotics that would improve the immune system. Corn, soy and antibiotics became the winning combination for feeding animals. In 1950 Thomas Jukes and Robert Stokstad, made a discovery while working with vitamins in animal feed programs. They found that fermented ground water they were using to extract vitamin B12, also produced the antibiotic aureomycin. They found by accident that adding only 5 pounds of the antibiotic to a ton of animal feed they could accelerate the growth of the animal by 50%. Animals given the antibiotic in their feed reach mature weight in half the time. This revolutionized agriculture. Today scientists believe that the sub therapeutic use of antibiotics in animal feed has contributed greatly to the development of so-called Super Bugs. The Super Bugs are bacteria that have evolved strains that are immune to most antibiotics. Today, MRSA, methicilin resistant staphylococcus aureus, is killing more Americans than HIV/AIDS. Antibiotics and other pharmaceutical drugs are nonbiodegradable. Like thousands of other man made substances, if Nature did not make them She will not take them back. They remain in the environment. All of the antibiotics and other pharmaceutical drugs ever used are still with us in the water and soil. We have few studies on the effects antibiotic residues might have on our body. We have to assume that our important symbiotic bacteria will be impacted in some way by exposure to antibiotics whether we take them directly or whether we are exposed through food or water. The Union of Concerned Scientists estimates that 25 million pounds of antibiotics are used in animal feed each year and that only about 3 million pounds are used for human medical needs. Despite the use of antibiotics, irradiation and other steps used by meat processors, thousands of people fall ill from salmonella, campylobacter and E. Coli each year. Meat and vegetable recalls are common place and more frequent than ever. Even casual surveys of food items show that drug resistant strains of bacteria are coming to market. Many childhood conditions including asthma and allergies are being connected to the sterile environment created from the over use of antibiotic medications and household products.

BULKING UP WITH HORMONES

In recent years growth hormones were added to improve weight gain. The hormones were also added to dairy feed to increase production. Today, corn, soy and antibiotics combine to make the feed given to cows, chickens, pigs, sheep and farm-raised fish. That is why I say that when you eat these animal products, you are also eating second hand corn and soy. The effects on the human body are further complicated by the hormones and the antibiotics. If it makes the cow fat, what will it do for those who eat the cow? The most common growth hormone is rBGH. It was produced by Monsanto by genetically modifying the anthrax bacteria. It is banned in every industrialized nation except the United States, Mexico and Brazil. rBGH increases estrogen. Studies show that animals that are given the growth hormone experience more cancers and other conditions directly related to estrogen balance. Studies show that children eating burgers made from meat of animals given rBGH experience hormonal imbalance. Some scientists believe the rBGH residue in meat and dairy products is one of the estrogen factors contributing to early sexual development. In 1991, President George Bush Sr. appointed Margaret Miller deputy director of the FDA. Among her first acts of office was the approval of rBGH to increase milk production. Prior to her appointment to the FDA Margaret Miller worked for Monsanto. She was a lead scientist in the development of rBGH. Yes, she approved her own work. One might say she was totally familiar with the program and totally qualified to make the decision, one might also say there was a blatant conflict of interest. The Margaret Miller story is not a rare occurrence. It is common for the FDA to have top appointments of people from the private sector with a clear conflict of interest.

One report states that an eight year old who eats two burgers from a drive thru restaurant will have a 25% hormonal imbalance because of the estrogen in the meat from the rBGH. Some scientists believe that the estrogen from the growth hormone and estrogens from environmental exposure to plastics are leading to hormonal changes in young people. Boys and girls are entering puberty at earlier ages each year. Some have anecdotally addressed the growing similarities between males and females in younger generations. Our bodies function and react to hormones. If we are bombarding our bodies with substances that mimic these hormones we cannot escape confusion and dysfunction of those systems that rely on them.

HIGH FAT – HIGH FRUCTOSE CORN SYRUP

Another leading cause of obesity is High Fructose Corn Syrup. It is another product made from corn. It is sweeter than sugar, it is easier to store, and it is easier to mix into products of all kinds. It is also cheaper than sugar. Politically, it provides a sweetener that does not require trade with Cuba, a leading producer of sugar. For the food and beverage industries HFCS is a winner. As far as taste goes, it is a winner for the consumer also. However, when the body tries to metabolize HFCS, a cascade of events is set off that results in fat making and can lead to insulin resistance and diabetes. Sugar is a twelve-carbon molecule. Glucose is a six-carbon molecule. When we ingest sugar the twelve-carbon molecule splits. The first six carbons convert to glucose. The second six-carbons become fruit sugar and also convert to glucose. This is why sugar produces twice the glucose than the amount produced by fructose, or fruit sugar. This is why candy is twice as fattening as fruit. However, when we juice the fruit, we concentrate the fructose and the body has a more difficult time with the unbound fructose. When we eat an apple, orange or other fruit, the fruit sugar is bound to the fiber. There are thousands of parents who control their children's intake of soda, and think it is OK to let them have all the juice they want. Juice in excess also can contribute to obesity and other health problems.

Unbound fructose interferes with some important hormones. It suppresses the production of insulin, it interferes with leptin and it stimulates the hunger hormone, ghrelin. The twelve-carbon HFCS molecule enters the body as half glucose and half unbound fructose. When we ingest HFCS we get a load of glucose that needs immediate insulin for conversion to energy in the cells. The HFCS suppression of insulin can contribute to insulin resistance and eventually type two diabetes. The glucose will probably convert to fat because of the impact HFCS has on leptin, the hormone that controls fat making among other body functions. Leptin is also a trigger for puberty. I personally would not be surprised to learn that early or pernicious puberty is often related to a child's intake of HFCS. The release of ghrelin in the stomach sends a hunger message to the brain. Consuming HFCS interferes with conversion of glucose to energy, stimulates fat making and causes hunger for more food than the body needs. How can we not question the relationship between HFCS and obesity. Since it began to replace sugar as the sweetener of choice in sodas and other beverages and thousands of sweet foods, we have seen obesity rise in the population.

FAT MAKING ADDITIVES

Another major fat maker is MSG, monosodium glutamate. The Japanese developed MSG as a food additive. It enhances the flavors of foods of all kinds. Restaurants use it to make stale salads taste fresh or to revive leftovers. I remember years ago when every kitchen had a shaker of Accent that was used to enhance the flavors of foods. It was also widely used as a meat tenderizer. The public has become more aware of the use of MSG and its undesirable side effects. Many people suffer from headaches after eating Chinese food that is frequently prepared with MSG. Proponents of MSG point out that it is essentially an amino acid, glutamate. If it is a natural body substance, how they ask, can it be harmful? Glutamine is a vital substance as a neurotransmitter. MSG loads the body with far more glutamine than is needed for neurotransmissions. It is among several substances including some artificial sweeteners used in the production of food that are classified as excitotoxins. These substances stimulate the nerves to carry messages from the brain. However, when the body is loaded with these substances, they over excite the brain or nerve cells and can actually cause them to burst. Some make things happen and some stop things from happening in the nerves that control our bodies. Glutamine is one of the substances that shuts things down. When we get an excess of glutamine from ingesting MSG, a Chinese food headache may be expected. The government classifies MSG as a condiment similar to salt and pepper. For those who have had bad reactions to MSG reading labels will not always protect them from it. MSG is a hidden ingredient in hundreds of foods because it can be listed under more than a dozen other names. I will leave the subject of MSG by telling you that it can be found in almost all processed foods, including drinking water, and

that when scientists want to conduct studies of obesity with rats, they give them MSG and they pack on the weight.

I am happy to see diet sodas listed among items that can contribute to obesity. Aspartame, the most common sugar substitute, is another excitotoxin. Aspartic acid is a neurotransmitter than makes things move. Excessive use is associated with seizures and neuromuscular disorders that often mimic diseases. Recent studies show that aspartame actually triggers cravings for carbohydrates and is now associated with obesity.

OVER FED AND MALNOURISHED

Our diet lacks the nutrients needed for good health including those needed for proper bone mass to avoid osteoporosis. I have only skimmed the surface of the adulteration of our food, I hope sufficiently to show a relationship between our diet and our declining health as a nation. Osteoporosis is one of several conditions made worse by the lack of nutrition in the food available to us through normal channels. There are some adulterations that have a specific impact on bone loss. One of the functions of a healthy skeleton is to serve as a storehouse for calcium and other minerals that can be leeched as needed to maintain balance in our bodies. For example, we release calcium to maintain a proper pH balance.

Anybody with experience maintaining a swimming pool is familiar with pH, potential for Hydrogen. It is the balance between acid and alkaline. Anybody who has tried to clear up a green swimming pool knows that the chemicals will not work if the pH is not in range. The human body functions best with a pH reading of 7.2 on a scale of zero to fourteen. When our system becomes too acid, it is more difficult to deliver vital oxygen to the cells. The skeleton responds by releasing calcium as an alkalizing agent. If a person has a high acid diet, the body will be burdened to release a greater amount of calcium to maintain pH balance. This can lead to a deficit of bone mass, or osteoporosis.

The standard American diet is filled with acid forming foods and beverages. Processing increases the acid content of even some foods that would normally be considered alkaline forming. The greater the amount of processed food in the diet the greater the probability for bone loss. Wheat becomes more acidic when the germ and bran are removed in the production of white flour. This process also reduces the bone building magnesium content to only a small amount. Soda made with HFCS is off the chart for high acid. It takes several glasses of water to neutralize the acid from a single soda. When one considers the amount of soda consumed by the average American woman each day, it is obvious that there is a connection to her bone loss.

While the acid in soda could be a leading cause of bone loss among American women, there is another negative impact on the skeleton. The body seeks to maintain balance among several minerals, including calcium and phosphorous. Soda contains a high amount of phosphorous and can cause calcium to leech from the bones to keep a proper ratio between them.

MUNICIPAL WATER SUPPLIES

AND BONE HEALTH

There are a number of studies showing a relationship between the consumption of fluoride and bone break from osteoporosis. Areas where public water supplies have been treated with fluoride tend to produce more cases of bone break from bone loss. Apparently, while fluoride can buildup calcium on the outer surface of a tooth, it may also similarly build on the inner surface of the tooth or bone cutting off the supply of nutrients. We have a new industry today for tooth whitening. Even chain operations in shopping malls are cashing in on the tooth whitening craze. People had white teeth before fluoride. Fluoride is a toxic waste material from the production of aluminum and other industrial operations. It was too toxic to dump into the environment, but OK for our children and our water supplies. The problems with the consumption of fluoride have been known for at least half of my more than 70 years. Why are municipalities still treating drinking water with it?

BONES AND SUNSHINE

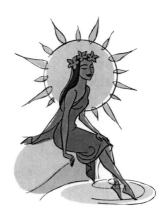

The link between vitamin D3 and healthy bone mass is
well established. This hormone-like vitamin is needed for
the body to produce and maintain healthy bones. Vitamin
D3 is the "sunshine vitamin". Through a process of
photosynthesis we make this vitamin from cholesterol.
Yes, cholesterol is important for making vitamin D3.
People with darker pigments in their skin actually require
more sunlight that those with more fair complexions to
make the vitamin. There is a link between bone break
from osteoporosis and geography. People in colder
climates that receive less full sun per year tend to have
less vitamin D3 than those living closer to the equator.
Our indoor lifestyle also creates a challenge to our
vitamin D3 stores. Another, more recent problem arises
from the use of sun screen lotions and other products that
keep the UV rays from the skin. These sun screens

reduce the production of vitamin D3 and probably contribute to bone loss, or the reduced ability to repair or make new bone mass.

Those who depend on milk for their vitamin D3 should know that dairy products are fortified with synthetic forms of vitamin D and that they can have limited if any positive impact on bone mass. They might also be disappointed to learn that calcium rich dairy products are not necessarily the bone builders we once thought they were. In fact, there are many nutritional scientists who now believe that excessive amounts of dairy might actually damage bone mass by forcing the body to surrender magnesium to maintain a balance with the calcium. And, it is doubtful that the calcium from pasteurized dairy, or other sources actually gets utilized in formulating the bone matrix by our bodies.

Another consideration for consuming dairy is the use of estrogenic growth hormones in its production. Meat and dairy farms have little restrictions on their use of growth hormones. Cattle add pounds and dairy cows produce more milk when they are given these hormones. There is a close link between estrogen and healthy bone mass. If there is a connection between the rising number of cases of osteoporosis and the use of estrogenic hormones in meat and dairy, it should be publicized. To say there is no connection is folly without studies. Again the regulators say there is no danger because the industry said there is no danger.

This is not a textbook and I offer no bibliography, although I do site my sources of information. This is not intended to be an expose on the harmful side of our pop-cuisine. While diet is a root cause of osteoporosis and other diseases, I am more interested in exposing you to the importance of the energetic science of nutrition.

My goal with this book is to stimulate more thought of what happens when the digestive enzymes and symbiotic flora realign the protons, neutrons and other components of the atoms in a food. There is a release of energy beyond our conventional concept of burning calories, or converting our food to glucose as fuel. I want us to begin to understand what Einstein meant when he said, "It is all energy." Perhaps when we understand more about the energy, we can begin to understand the Supreme Intelligence he described as the next step beyond energy.

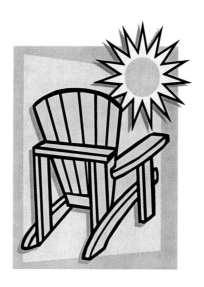

HOW IMPORTANT ARE CALCIUM SUPPLEMENTS?

Excessive use of calcium supplements may actually disrupt the body's ability to formulate bone. This might explain why people with excellent bone mineral density readings are among the first to suffer a broken bone. It is pretty clear that the calcium we are using in supplements and to fortify everything from soda and candy bars to orange juice has not changed the prediction that half the women over 50 years of age will experience a bone break from osteoporosis at least once in her life time. I have come to believe that humans and other mammals do not absorb dietary calcium in sufficient amounts for maintaining bone mass. Calcium is an essential nutrient for vegetation. Calcium in the soil produces magnesium in the fruits and vegetables. Magnesium and other minerals are biologically transmuted in our bodies to make the calcium we need for bone mass.

The latest studies show that we can absorb and use only about 500 mg of calcium citrate per day. With normal consumption of dairy and leafy greens we should have more than 1000 mg total calcium intake from our diets. More and more the evidence appears to be telling us that the amount of calcium is not as important as the form of the calcium in our diet. Also, it appears that the recent studies are pointing to how the body processes the calcium and other minerals needed for the bone matrix. While the bone contains calcium carbonate, this appears to be the least absorbable form. The carbonate apparently forms a sludge with stomach acids. This may be an effective antacid, but not a desirable nutrient for bone health. Healthy gut flora may be more important for the support of bone mass, than the calcium and other nutrients in our diet. If we do not have the components for good digestion in place, our good diet may be wasted or ineffective.

CALCIUM, THE SUPPLEMENT

I am not a fan of the current trend of publishing a statistical analysis of previous studies, as a study. The results are easily manipulated, and one can draw conclusions of convenience if they have a particular point to make. It is possible to support a product or a conclusion without ever actually putting it to the test. The statistical result of an analysis of scientific studies is actually no stronger than a collection of anecdotal experiences. The original study may have been double-blind and scientific, but the "science" does not extend to the analytical evaluation. Often these profiles are published in respected journals and passed off as scientific studies.

A few of these kinds of articles have been published concerning calcium. Most were slanted to support a particular form of calcium supplement. Other similar type studies have found that taking calcium had no impact on bone mass. It is tempting to include some of these reports to support my case against massive calcium supplementation, but I will refrain.

There are some valid studies that are worthy of consideration in this text. The Harvard Nurses Study has followed large numbers of people over a period of several years to track their health information. In this study, taking calcium supplements showed no significant relationship to bone mass. In other words, taking a daily calcium supplement did not improve bone mass.

Another important study came to a similar conclusion, The Woman's Health Initiative. This one involved a million women. It was cut short because it showed that estrogen and progestin actually caused some of the health problems they were supposed to prevent. The dangers of estrogen replacement therapy got the headlines, but the third phase of the study involved bone mass and calcium supplementation. Although the study was not completed because of the discoveries involving estrogen and progestin, the data that were compiled showed that taking calcium supplements did not improve bone mass.

The information available today is leading many experts to believe that calcium supplements might actually do more harm than good. Excessive amounts of calcium can cause muscle spasms, it can deposit in organs and tissues, make bone spurs or plaque in the walls of blood vessels or in kidneys, heart, and liver, and in some cases it might actually increase the risk of cancer. Other conditions include migraine headaches, joint and muscle pain, kidney stones, and even depression. Remember, Americans have the best bone density tests on the planet. Despite consuming milk and milk products and calcium supplements at one of the highest rates in the world, we still have among the highest rates of osteoporosis and bone break. Something is dreadfully wrong. .

MILKING THE ISSUE

We are taught at every level in our culture that milk provides calcium for the bones. We give it to our children and tell them they need it if they want to grow tall. As adults we are told to consume dairy products for calcium. We add it to orange juice and other beverages. I recently saw commercials for water with added calcium and at least one brand of soda offers calcium. The US Recommended Daily Allowance for calcium is as high as 1,200 milligrams for some age groups, plus several servings of dairy.

I am compelled to tell you at this point that I completely distrust the RDAs and other government policies and recommendations concerning food and supplements. Starting with the USDA Food Pyramid, recommendations concerning nutrition are not based on the needs of the consumers, but on the abundance of the products. We are told to eat and drink what the food producers need to sell. The regulatory agencies are devoted to promoting commerce, not protecting consumers. After spending millions of our tax dollars on a "price support" program that controls the milk industry at a surplus level of production, we are promoted to consume the milk and dairy products. Anybody with a few acres, a barn and a herd of cows can be a milk farmer. The government will buy the milk. It takes some expert know-how to make a living on what the government pays, but that is another issue. At least the milk farmer has a buyer for the product, the US

Government. That which is not consumed is made into powdered milk or phony cheese for storage. Some well connected individuals get paid handsomely for storing the excess product. Eventually the excess is sold at a cheap rate or given away at senior centers. All funded by tax dollars, not a free marketplace. With so much invested in milk and dairy products, little wonder why the USDA wants us to consume lots of dairy products daily.

Many studies, including the Harvard Nurses Study, show a relationship between dairy consumption and increased bone break. Yes, those who consumed the most dairy had the most bone breaks. Volumes could be written on the health conditions among children that can be traced to their consumption of milk. Even, Type One Diabetes, according to one recent report. Studies from Australia and New Zealand also show higher incidents of bone break among those who consume the most dairy products.

T. Colin Campbell, was raised on a dairy farm in Virginia. For years he not only consumed milk, but also believed the conventional wisdom that milk consumption produces strong bones. Experience as a researcher, including 10 years in China, convinced him that the conventional wisdom was flawed. Dr. Campbell believes that a mostly vegetarian diet with low animal protein consumption is the primary reason why those that do not consume milk products have a history of fewer bone breaks. These conclusions are in his book, *The China Study.* This book should be read by every parent and any other person in a position of planning menus for other people.

BIOLOGICAL TRANSMUTATION

OR COLD FUSION IN LIVING MATTER

"The serious error of scientists consists in their saying that reactions in living matter are solely chemical reactions, that chemistry can and must explain life".
Louis Kervran

"The experimental method consists in revising theorems and not in preserving them. Theory must adopt to nature but nature need not adapt to theory". Claude Bernard

Pasteur, on his death bed, confirmed to Renon: "Bernard was correct when he said: *'When one encounters a fact which conflicts with a dominant theory, one must accept the fact and abandon the theory, even though the latter is supported by influential people and widely accepted'.*

I have struggled with my thoughts for several weeks before beginning to draft this part of the book. First, I have worked to phrase my disclaimers, or explanations of why I think I might be able to explain something that I do not understand fully. Second, I wanted to review the material available on biological transmutation or "low energy transmutation". I will share some of the studies that make me secure in the validity of the phenomenon, but first let me present my disclaimers.

I am neither a chemist nor a physicist. Perhaps that makes it easy for me to embrace something that goes beyond the mainstream theories of both fields. I will not pretend to understand these disciplines on a molecular level, much less on an atomic, or isotopic level.

However, having seen the power of an atom bomb in my lifetime, I am not surprised to learn that there is extreme energy within the atom. In high school science we learn that the atom has protons and neutrinos. We see drawings that tell us the tiny atom is a miniature solar system. More advanced science would teach us about other components that have been identified in the last few years.

At the layman's level we can deal with some of the better known components. An atom is the smallest part of anything according to Webster:

at·om

Etymology:

> Middle English, from Latin *atomus,* from Greek *atomos,* from *atomos* indivisible, from *a-* + *temnein* to cut

1 : one of the minute indivisible particles of which according to ancient materialism the universe is composed 2 : a tiny particle : 3 : the smallest particle of an element that can exist either alone or in combination 4 : the atom considered as a source of vast potential energy

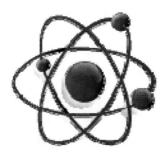

Atoms are made up of combinations of protons, electrons and usually, but not always, some neutrons. An isotope is a particular kind of atom.

iso·tope

Etymology:

  is- + Greek *topos* place

1 : any of two or more species of atoms of a chemical element with the same atomic number and nearly identical chemical behavior but with differing atomic mass or mass number and different physical properties.

The weight of each element is different depending on the number of protons and neutrons it has in an atom. The elements are arranged by their atomic number, which is the number of protons in that element. Also listed is that elements atomic weight, or the average number of protons and neutrons. If the number of protons was different, it would be a different element. The unit of atomic weight was fixed at 1/12 the atomic weight of a carbon atom. Most of us learned about protons, neutrons and electrons in high school or freshman science classes. The developing science of subatomic physics deals with far more than those three familiar components. Leptons, gluons, bosons, quarks and similar particles are among the components of the atoms. The idea of atoms giving up or gaining particles suddenly appears more feasible than the old concepts of Lavoisier. The Father of Chemistry believed and taught that an atom of a given element is absolute, and will always be what it is. Today, subatomic physicists have sophisticated equipment that can combine elements. One of the earliest was the combination of tin and copper that made gold.

With nuclear fission and fusion physicists routinely bombard and combine elements at their atomic level. The developing of isotopes is needed for the harnessing of nuclear power. But biological transmutation or low energy transmutation is not the same as fission or fusion. Creating an element from one or more other elements has been accomplished through fission and fusion with the application of extreme heat and pressure. In biological or low energy transmutation elements are created in living matter by hormones and enzymes. Scientists knew

68

something was happening for a very long time before they were able to offer reasonable explanations of the phenomenon. Today, it is clear that with an exchange or rearrangement of components within the atom, it is transmuted into a different element. Energy becomes matter, or matter becomes energy.

An atom remains the smallest particle of any given element. Subatomic matter goes into the basic soup that all elements come from. While an atom is the smallest particle of any given element, its subatomic particles can be increased or removed, in which case the atomic weight is different and it is an atom, or smallest particle of another element.

Although the science applied to biological transmutation exceeds the Einstein theory of relativity, we must honor his teachings on the nature of matter, "It is all energy, and beyond that Supreme Intelligence". It is within the atom that the scientist who is open can see the Intelligence of life and its creation. I will not attempt to settle any arguments in this work, but I will offer an opinion. I believe that too many scientists believe the world came out of chaos and that man has crafted order. I prefer to believe that the world was created by Intelligence and that man has brought chaos to natural harmony. This is the subject of my next book, and I have lots of homework to do before moving more deeply into the subject. By the way, Einstein never claimed his theory of relativity applied to living matter. Just for the record in case you are curious, I believe in evolution.

However, I believe that there is more to life and our process of "becoming" than being the most fit to survive. Survival fitness may influence our primal breeding instincts on the surface, but we are endowed with a deep need for concrescence, if I may borrow a term from the great Alfred North Whitehead. Intelligent Design is a more progressive Creationism; better than Darwin, but neither should be taught as scientific fact.

One of the quickest ways to begin to understand biological transmutation is the chicken and the egg.

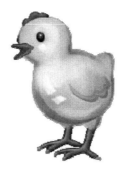

Without trying to prove which came first, it has been shown that the calcium in the egg is confined to the shell. The little chick hatches by breaking through the shell. It hatches with a strong beak and a skeleton, both of which contain calcium. The calcium did not come from the shell; therefore, it had to be biologically transmuted from the other elements that were in the egg.

The cow gives us an even better example. She gives many gallons of milk rich in calcium and does not suffer from osteoporosis. Adding calcium to her diet or

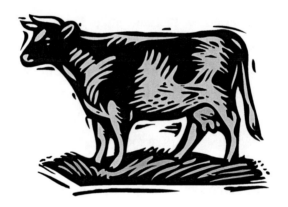

supplementing her diet with calcium does not have an impact on the amount of calcium in her milk or the amount of milk she produces. She depends on two main sources of food, grass and corn silage. The grass and the corn are rich in the magnesium she needs to make the calcium. The grass and the corn need calcium rich soil to deliver the magnesium needed to enrich the milk. If a farmer wants to keep his cow producing, he will add calcium in the form of limestone to the soil where the grass and corn are grown. Limestone in the soil increases the magnesium content of the plants. Magnesium increases the calcium content of the milk.

At our home, Pleasant Stone Farm, we have a large field that at one time was fenced and used as a paddock for our horses. The children moved away and we got tired of frozen water buckets and mucking stalls. When our last horse passed on at the age of 32, we took down the fencing and started mowing the field. It has beautiful turf. I thought the healthy grass came from years of horse droppings, but discovered that nature has her own way of taking care of harmony and balance. Each year in the spring the field is covered with daisies and buttercups. I mow around the flowers until their blossoms wither. I found out researching this book that daisies and buttercups enrich the soil with calcium. I never spread limestone. The beautiful grass comes from nature's own enrichment. I always thought that weeds and wild flowers grew where their seeds were carried by birds and the wind. I know now that nature plants what the soil needs. Any amateur gardener knows that virgin soil produces a fine first year garden, or that land that has been fallow for a couple of years has regained virgin status. Nature has her own way of harmonizing the soil if it is left alone.

Several strains of bamboo are known to enrich soil with calcium the same as crown vetch is often used to "fix" soil and protect its nitrogen content and micro organisms. We are engaged in chemical farming today. Our food production has become dependent on fossil fuel for artificial fertilizers and pesticides and herbicides. The more chemicals we use, the more chemicals we need to produce food. Finally, science is beginning to understand that chemicals are not good for our bodies. At one time it was claimed that chemically synthesized substances were the same as natural substances. Today, it is shown that there is a major difference even if the chemical substance does have the same formula as the natural one. Rudolf Steiner introduced "balanced agriculture" in the 1920s. In ancient Peru in an area that may have been the site of the fabled Atlantis, irrigation ditches remain from a time when food was produced in great abundance. We are much too quick to think that the mainstream is the best we can do. We can no longer ignore the biological transmutations that take place in all living matter, if we are to move away from the health crisis we have created.

In the 17th century von Helmont planted a tree in 200 pounds of soil. Five years later he had a 160 pound tree and the container lost only 2 ounces of soil. Where did 160 pounds of bark, wood and leaves come from? We may not have the answer to that question even today. We do know a great deal more about photosynthesis today, and we know without a doubt that elements are not absolute in living matter.

As early as 1799 French chemist, Vuequelin studied the amount of limestone, or calcium carbonate produced by laying hens every day. He found that the hens gave up far more calcium than they consumed.

It was an English physiologist, Prout who did the studies on the hatching chicks which developed a skeleton without taking calcium from the shell of the egg. That was in 1822.

Magnesium + oxygen = calcium
Potassium + hydrogen = calcium
Silica + carbon = calcium

It was French scientist, Louis Kervran who devoted his career to experiments and data expanding and proving the theories of biological transmutation. He found that hydrogen and oxygen were the mediators, along with carbon. Kervran carried out countless experiments on the phenomenon. He also gathered the findings of others on the subject for his books and papers. He was published in French and the books are out of print. They can still be obtained by used book vendors and several online book sellers. There is considerable and reliable information supporting biological transmutation on the internet.

WHAT DOES ALL THIS HAVE TO DO WITH OSTEOPOROSIS?

We are mammals, much like the cow. There are many established parallels in nutrition between people and the bovine. We certainly devour thousands of gallons of milk in the United States. We are one of the very few societies that uses milk as a food after weaning from breast milk. Milk is promoted as a food source of calcium. Well, perhaps we have more in common with the cow that we thought. Perhaps, we too do not get our calcium directly from the diet. There is good reason to believe that we do not absorb dietary calcium. The prediction that one in every two women over fifty years of age will suffer a fracture from osteoporosis is pretty solid evidence that something in our system does not work. We consume plenty of dairy in this country. We take tons of calcium supplements. We still have a serious health threat from bone loss.

I have often been critical of the "statistical analysis of previous studies" because one can tweak statistics to conclude convictions held prior to the start of the analysis. In other words, such a study can prove just about anything the sponsors hope to prove. If the study is sponsored by a supplement company, it probably concludes that supplements make a difference. The Dairy Council has proved the value of dairy products and pharmaceuticals can prove the value of bone building medications. A simple review of previous studies however, can also show that supplements and dairy products have little if any impact on bone mass. There are several studies that found no impact from supplements among older subjects. One study suggested that taking calcium supplements would reduce osteoporosis in an additional five women per 10,000. It also showed however, that it would increase by five per 10,000 the number of women who would have kidney stones from the calcium. I have followed the studies and reports in the major journals for several years and have found more reports that show little or no effect from calcium supplements than reports that show significant improvements.

The cutting edge of modern nutrition remarkably cuts the RDA for calcium by at least half, no more than 500 mg of calcium citrate or similar form. The RDA for vitamin D has been increased to 800 iu. The modern nutritionist would suggest at least 1,000 iu of vitamin D.

If you want more information on biological transmutation, see the reference material at the end of the book. I have not burdened you with countless examples of this phenomenon. It comes down to expanding Lavoisier's laws in biochemistry. The statement that "Nothing is lost, nothing is created" can apply universally to dead matter. It cannot apply to living matter, however. The belief that H2O, water is always water, whether in solid, liquid or gaseous form does not apply to living matter. If it did you could soak a raisin in water and get a grape. You get a plump raisin, but it will never again be a grape. More than water is lost in the drying process. Actually, the belief that water remains water in living matter is an assumption, not a fact.

Lavoisier was a great scholar of the 18th century. He is called the father of modern chemistry. The atom is said to be the smallest part of anything, and if it should become separated from the two or more atoms needed to form a molecule, it would be found in another molecule. This was the law and there was no discussion. Marie

Curie broke new ground for thought in the 20th century when she discovered that some radioactive elements transmute into other elements. The alchemists of the 17th century were ridiculed for their beliefs from the Middle Ages. Today Lavoisier's law is still taught in university chemistry and physics classes. But on the cutting edge of nutrition and biochemistry it is accepted today that there is activity in the energy of the atom. The atoms give up or accept components from other atoms to form different elements.

I can easily believe that Helmont's 160 pound tree was grown from hydrogen and oxygen from H2O that was transmuted into other elements in the living matter. Why not theorize that the oxygen needed to make calcium from magnesium can come from water. Or why not theorize that the hydrogen needed to make calcium from potassium comes from H2O.

The sea creatures that form shells for protection have virtually no calcium in their diet or available to them in their environment. They take magnesium, plentiful in seawater, and transmute it into calcium carbonate for their shells. There was a very active marketing program promoting Coral Calcium. Coral Calcium comes from the discarded shells of sea creatures harvested from the ocean floor or beach sand. However, it is just limestone and no more bioavailable than other forms of carbon calcinate. Kervran theorizes beyond living matter. He thinks the earth's deposits of coal and oil may not have come from vegetation or animals. He believes that the elements gained sulfur from other elements and pressure under the earth's crust to form the deposits of "fossil fuel". They may not be fossilized after all. This would explain why some geologists date oil and coal deposits older than life forms. It could also explain the oil and coal deposits in the frozen arctic regions as well as the arid deserts where vegetation and animal life would have been difficult to sustain.

AGAIN, WHAT DOES ALL THIS HAVE TO DO WITH BONE MASS?

Perhaps we should supplement with magnesium and vitamin D. We also know that the silica in the herb, horsetail, builds healthy bone and speeds healing from fractures. Perhaps, dairy with its calcium content is not the answer, nor are the calcium supplements being taken in large amounts.

My wife and many of the people who seek my counsel for their health and nutrition have been taking magnesium, vitamin D and horsetail for many months.

All are getting good Bone Mineral Density Tests and not one is a candidate for the bone building medications. I also urge them to eat fresh greens daily for the vitamin K. Other minerals and vitamins are important for bone mass, but they are found in a good multivitamin and mineral complex and a well rounded diet.

I have used horsetail for many years in support of healthy bones. Especially, when people have had broken bones, I mixed them a tisane with horsetail, boneset and other herbs. Their doctors were always surprised at how quickly their bones would heal. I also urged them to hold a cat and allow it to purr. The purring of a cat matches the vibration used in a Brown University study that showed increased electromagnetic activity around bone breaks when the treatments were applied.

 Dr. Earl Staelin writing in a 2008 edition of *The Journal of Well Being* relates some case histories from his practice showing that horsetail, or silicon improved the bone health of his patients. In fact, his article, "Strong Bones or Osteoporosis, Part I: Beware of Too Much Calcium" offers strong support for the positions I am taking in this work.

"It is very clear that bacteria have been here much longer than we have, and that as far as they're concerned, we may just be a passing feature in their history."

Dr. Stuart Levy, M.D., 2000

OUR UNSEEN SYMBIOTS

Long before God brought us out of the sea and long before we walked on the Earth, He made microbes to help prepare the environment for our existence and survival. We could not experience life as we know it on our planet without the symbiotic relationships between microbes and larger organisms. From releasing nitrogen for the roots of plants to digesting food in the stomach of a mammal, microbes are an important and irreplaceable part of our lives and the life around us. Microbiology and subatomic physics are the new frontiers of learning in the twenty first century. These two disciplines, perhaps more than any others, can provide a platform where science communicates with intelligence and where energy is defined for mortal comprehension.

Osteoporosis is one of the many metabolic conditions that can be alleviated with a better understanding of the bonds between our bodies and the Earth. As I will say many times, "Malnutrition is the root cause of metabolic disease". The human body is a little over six pounds of Earth, or elements, and the remainder is sea water or saline. We came from the Earth and our food choices are supposed to keep us bonded to the Earthly Mother. Proper diet is also, in most cases, capable of reversing conditions of illness if the subject has not exceeded the body's natural ability to restore or heal itself. The two ingredients missing from most therapies are the most vital ones for healing: energy and intelligence, both of which are found in whole foods. Modern science is telling us what our Faith told us years earlier, that every atom is energy and every atom of living matter has intelligence. Biological transmutation has shown us that atoms of living matter can use intelligence to change and adjust the energetics of their composition. This process takes place with the help of symbiotic microbes. Is there communication between the intelligence of the atoms of living matter and the intelligence of symbiotic microbes? I would think that after all these years of cohabitation they would have overcome their language barriers to facilitate an exchange of information.

MICROBIAL INTELLIGENCE

If we rake off the newly fallen leaves from the forest floor and reach for a handful of the richly organic soil, we will be holding thousands of little creatures. These microbes are engaged in nurturing our planet and our lives. If we take a swab of saliva from our mouth we can find as many as 400 different species of microbes. Most of these, along with hundreds more in our digestive tract, are engaged in nurturing number of the millions of microbes or germs found in our environment are capable of causing illness. Many times these disease causing microbes can make us ill, only because we are lacking the so-called good germs or microbes that would have neutralized them on contact. A major portion of our immune response capability consists of gut flora, intestinal microbes, which have a symbiotic relationship with us as their host. All microbes demonstrate a sense of community and an intelligence that goes beyond Darwinian survival impulses. Even at the beginning of our lives we are protected by microbes. As the fetus makes its way to the open air of the delivery room, the birth canal is coated with a slick lubricant that is filled with good microbes. They immediately die when exposed to the oxygen rich air, but in their death they produce a form of peroxide that protects the tender skin of the newborn baby from infection and harm. For me this is another example of Creative Intelligence. For the scientist it is a demonstration of another symbiotic relationship between organisms and microbes.

"What unifying force drives the behavior of all living systems? Pose this question to a dozen biologists and the same answer will emerge: survival. In the mainstream view, life exists solely for it own perpetuation. This view strikes me as needlessly nihilistic-and on deeper analysis, wrong."
Dr. Frank T. Vertosick, Jr., *The Genius Within*

When the baby penguins are ready for the first fishing trip into the icy ocean waters, years of evolution tell them that sea lions are in the water waiting to end their short lives. One penguin will pick a spot and enter the water. If bloody foam erupts the penguins on shore know that this is not the spot to enter the water. If nothing happens, they know that there are no sea lions or other predators waiting for them and that it is a safe place to enter the water. For the first penguin entering the water, it could be a lucky day or a violent death. The driving force behind this penguin's behavior clearly, is not survival, at least not solely its own. This behavior demonstrates a desire for community or concrescence, if you will.

Among the microbes we find a deep commitment to community and group or species survival. Truly it is all for one and one for all in this setting. Let us look at the disease causing germs and what these microbes have revealed about themselves in the last half century, following the introduction of antibiotic medications.

There are two kinds of microbes: prokaryotic and eukaryotic. Procaryotes (pro-carry-oats) have no nucleus or membrane enclosed structure. They are the most common type of bacteria. Eukaryotes (u-carry-oats) include plants, animals, fungi and microbic parasites. Both have cell or plasma membrane enclosures. Eukaryotes have a nucleus and a variety of internal structures known as organelles, "little organs", which are also surrounded by membranes. Microbes have DNA and chromosomes which are passed along in duplication of new generations. Most antibiotics work by blocking replication or by dissolving the membrane encasement.

A BRIEF HISTORY OF MEDICINE

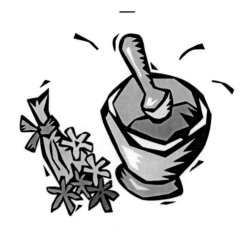

2000 B.C.E – "Here, eat this root".
1000 A.D – "The root is heathen. Here, say this prayer".
1850 – "That prayer is superstitious. Here, drink this potion".
1920 – "That portion is snakeoil. Here, swallow this pill".
1945 – "That pill is ineffective. Here, take this penicillin".
1955 - "Oops, bugs got resistant. Here, take this tetracycline".
1957 – 2007 "Oops x 42. Here, take this more powerful antibiotic".
2008 - :The germs have won. Here, eat this root."

Anonymous

In 1928 Sir Alexander Fleming, a microbiologist at St. Mary's Hospital in London, noticed that his staphylococcal cultures were not growing in the presences of a mold that had contaminated some of the dishes. He identified the mold as *penicillin,* a microbe found in soil. Years later a team of doctors at Oxford led by Howard Florey working with an American pharmaceutical firm devised a way of refining it for safe delivery to patients. The age of antibiotics began. By 1941 the scientific community was congratulating its superior brain power for overcoming the lowly infectious germs that caused disease. By 1942 they were taking note of resistance among germs that were displaying an ability to survive *penicillin.* The drug worked by blocking the germ's ability to reproduce or form new cells. It was only effective against cells undergoing division. It was not attracted to resting cells. Some cells learned to play dead to avoid the effects of *penicillin.* Soon bacteria discovered that by producing an enzyme called lactamases they could interfere with the betalactam ring of the *penicillin* molecule and render it ineffective. It was the beginning of bacteria mutating to become immune to antibiotics. The bacteria can swap DNA with other bacteria, it can exchange chromosomes, and it can attach viruses to itself to accelerate its mutations. Microbes can fast track these changes and experience several generations of change in a matter of hours. What we learned from antibiotic resistance among bacteria is that there is a community intelligence that so far has out performed the best scientific minds of the pharmaceutical community.

As scientific efforts to control infection moved from *penicillin* to ever stronger forms of antibiotics, it became evident that microbes were much more than celibate, asexual loners making their way through evolution with occasional mutations. For germs to develop the ability to produce lactamases they had to reach into other species and go back many generations. Microbes showed themselves to be a close working community with the ability to transfer information and genetic material across species in a short period of linear development. Mammals can take years to evolve a particular genetic trait. Microbes can evolve new genetic traits very quickly, in hours or days.

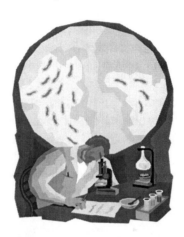

As I write this in 2008 my mother-in-law who is ninety-two and in a nursing home has been isolated because she has developed a drug resistant *E. coli* urinary infection. This afternoon I heard a radio report of concerns in London because of the many cases of drug resistant Tuberculosis being carried by travelers. I myself carry MRSA, *methicillin*-resistant-*Staph. Arereus,* from a hospital infection. Daily we hear about germs and viruses that no longer respond to the most common medications. Microbes, single cell life forms without a brain, are displaying an intelligence that is baffling our best brains in medical science.

In all fairness, not all of the blame for the evolvement of the so-called "superbugs" can be placed on the antibiotics used to treat human infections. In 1950 two employees of a pharmaceutical giant discovered that putting a small amount of antibiotics in animal feed caused the animals to reach their mature weight in less time. Although the use of antibiotics for farm animals is being reduced today, the tons of antibiotics used in

animal feed far exceed the amount used to treat humans. Due to a massive public education campaign, we finally know that antibiotics do nothing for infections not caused by bacteria, and doctors are prescribing fewer antibiotics. Another culprit is our inbred fear of microbes. Actually, researchers are finding that many allergies and similar conditions among children can develop from not being exposed to microbes. We have tried to kill all the bad germs, but we may have made them stronger. And we may have killed as many good germs as bad. A bad germ is still a bad germ, but we cannot live a healthy life without the good germs. As a result of our use of antibiotics and germ killing agents, we have filled our soil and waters with them. They have passed through the humans and animals to remain in our environment for a very long time. So, even though we are reducing the use of these compounds, we can still experience the side effects from environmental exposure.

NOW THE GOOD NEWS

You may be asking why I am writing about infections in a book about a metabolic condition. I am using the ability of the infectious microbes to demonstrate the fact that they act as a community, all for one and one for all, and that they have intelligence to do so. Now the good news:

they symbiotic microbes in our body and every cell of our body have the same intelligence. We may have been so impressed with our brain power that we overlooked what ancient healers knew about the energy and intelligence of the human body. We are beginning to return to the power of thought, prayer, visualization and faith in treating the conditions that do not respond to our best medications.

As I said in a previous section, we have no single organ devoted to our immune system. The bone marrow is the source of many of the components the body uses to neutralize invaders. We have a cascade of events in response to germs that get into our bodies. We send out warrior antibodies to block them, histamine to surround them, a rise in temperature to control them. It is a regular crime scene in our body. Special cells show up like a CSI team to take photos and collect DNA samples. This information is on file and should the same, or even similar, bacteria come back into the neighborhood, the Swat Team is ready and can quickly identify the trouble makers. This is intelligence equal to the smarts the bad guys use to avoid our antibiotics.

We not only have an intelligent immune system at work inside our bodies; but also an intelligent team working outside, our symbiots, the millions of microbes in our mouth and digestive and elimination tract. Think of the body as having a tube running through it from the lips to the end of the colon. It is about thirty feet long. Most of it coiled as the large intestine. When we chew our food and swallow, it is still outside the body and passing through this tube. Chewing prepares the food for digestion. We secrete hydrochloric acid to sterilize it in the stomach.

We secrete other enzymes depending on what we have sent down to be digested. These digestive enzymes are guided by an intelligence of the body that has determined by taste and texture what will be needed to process the food, and also what the body needs most to extract from it. The next step in digestion is the work of the microbes. Just like the microbes that are preparing organic material for the roots of trees in the forest, our gut flora will work our food into small particles that can pass through the gut wall and reach the liver. In the liver the food is loaded on little trucks of LDL cholesterol for delivery to every cell.

Our digestion is similar to a septic system. Solid matter coming into the septic tank from the house is worked into a liquid form by bacteria. The liquid is displaced by new solids entering the tank and it flows into a leach field where it vaporizes. The solids we have ingested have to be worked into a liquid before they enter the body, and that is the work of our good gut flora, our symbiotic microbes. There is still another display of intelligence in the digestive process. Somehow, the colony of digestive microbes will know what might be missing from the food that is needed by the body, B vitamins for example. The gut flora can make B vitamins. Gut flora also makes vitamin K and other nutrients. It is logical to assume that this is the place where biological transmutations

Begin to take place in the human body. We know that the osteoblasts are formed in the digestive tract for delivery to the bones. The osteoblast contains all of the components of healthy bone. It is the osteoblast that will replace the bone that is lost in the form of osteoclasts. It is normal to lose or surrender bone for all the reasons we have discussed earlier. When there is a deficit in replacing the bone mass, osteoporosis develops.

There are few studies on the work of digestive microbes in humans. The literature is filled with information on the digestive workings of cows and the role of microbes. The mainstream view of human digestion, however, relies on the chemicals secreted by the body and the work of the liver. Little is known with certainty about the role of our gut flora. We do know for sure after a dose of antibiotics that digestion suffers and the bowel is irregular. We also know that antibiotic use can lead to a yeast overgrowth or infection because the normal gut flora is not in place to control the fungal growth.

Whether biological transmutation takes place within the microbial colony of our digestive system or in the liver, or whether they both share the chore, we must accept the proven theory that it is taking place. All other living matter demonstrates biological transmutation, why not humans?

Louis Kervran believed that the only a small amount of calcium could be metabolized by the human body. That small amount would be needed for cardio vascular health and muscle tone. He believed, and proved, that bone support came from the transmutation of magnesium, potassium, or silica into bone matrix or osteoblasts. Obviously, the catalyst that causes biological transmutations in living matter is intelligence. Then it is clear, that good digestion depends on gut flora, and that control of osteoporosis and other metabolic diseases begins with our intelligent hidden symbiots. It remains our responsibility to limit or remove from our diet the substances that might impede this process, and to include the substances that will support our nutritional needs. In addition to a well rounded all natural diet, I would include 400 to 800 mg of Magnesium, 1000 mg of horsetail and 1000 iu of vitamin D3. Plus zinc, boron and vitamin.

MINERALS AND OTHER IMPORTANT NUTRIENTS

CALCIUM

I believe we could spend the next ten years going over the calcium studies that are available, and design and carry out some new ones, without clearing the confusion surrounding dietary calcium. I have seen a pattern. Studies that were connected to a specific product tend to support its use. More wide open studies tend to show no benefits from calcium supplements or consumption of dairy in maintaining bone mass. Studies that do show marked improvement in bone mass are those that involve other minerals and nutrients, with or without calcium.

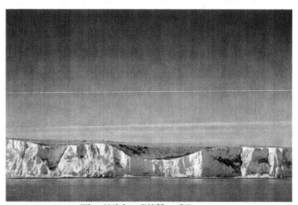

The White Cliffs of Dover

Calcium is one the most plentiful minerals in the crust of our Earthly Mother. The famous White Cliffs of Dover, for example, are limestone or calcium carbonate. We have already discussed the importance of limestone in agriculture to sweeten or alkalize the soil. Plants also transmute the calcium in the soil to magnesium.

While there are limited studies showing the dangers of excessive intake of calcium there is at least mounting speculation that it can be harmful. It is doubtful that such a study will be funded in the near future because there would be no way to profit from it. Profits and patents are the only reasons for funding a scientific study. Even studies funded by the government from tax dollars are somehow tied to the marketplace.

When we take a close look at studies that show improvement of bone mass among a significant number of participants, we invariably find that nutrients other than calcium were involved. The use of Microcrystaline calcium hydroxyapatite had been shown to improve bone mass. MCHA as we pointed out earlier is made from calf bone and has the proper ratio of elements in addition to the calcium. We do not know with certainty whether the body digests and uses MCHA, or whether it dismantles it and utilizes the support minerals or the calcium to produce the osteoblasts. Again, we do know that there are good results among those who have been given those other minerals.

We cannot ignore the quality of bone in determining its strength. We base our assessments of osteoporosis solely on bone mass as measured by one of the BMD tests. We know that people with the most bone mass are often those with the most bone breaks. We are compelled to assume that these people have a mass of bone that is missing important components of strength. Asian women with extremely thin bones in their advancing years, seldom experience an osteoporotic bone break.

It would be folly to suggest that no dietary calcium be consumed. We need calcium for use in our body for functions other than maintaining a healthy skeleton. Our muscle tone depends on calcium, so does our cardio vascular system. Still, there is a growing consensus among those who are close to the situation suggesting that the RDA for calcium be reduced. This is probably a first. Usually those close to emerging scientific nutritional data are calling for increases in the RDAs. Most appear to agree that calcium should be cut by at least half to 400 mg to 500 mg of supplemental calcium per day. There appears to be nothing to support the fortification of foods and beverages with calcium. While calcium obviously is important for healthy bones, it appears that the body prefers to make its own from magnesium, potassium, or silica. We do know that the osteoblasts that are needed for the regeneration of skeletal bone are made in the digestive process. One vital component of the osteoblast is produced by our gut flora, Vitamin K. The liver completes their preparation for delivery to the bone.

Several recent studies have cast serious doubt on the consumption of animal protein and supplemental calcium. In addition to the work of T. Colin Campbell in *The China Study*, studies such as the European Prospective Investigation into Cancer and Nutrition link calcium from dairy products to cancer. The study collected data from 142,251 men over a period of 8.7 years. There was an increase in prostate cancer in relation to the amount of dairy products consumed. The authors concluded, "That a high intake of protein or calcium from dairy products may increase the risk of prostate cancer. Men are not normally associated with osteoporosis, and women certainly are not associated with prostate cancer. It does demonstrate reasonable doubt concerning the consumption of large amounts of "dairy for the bones".

MAGNESIIUM

Magnesium + Oxygen = Calcium

Magnesium may be the most costly deficiency in the American diet. Every condition from simple constipation to diabetes is influenced by the amount of this work horse mineral in the diet. Refining and processing of our foods greatly reduces the amount of magnesium content. I cannot recall ever seeing or hearing about a product that was fortified with magnesium. In fact, because magnesium is a rather large molecule most manufacturers limit the amount they put into their multi vitamin and mineral tablets.

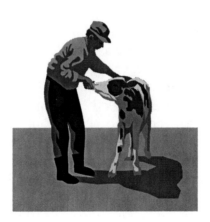

In 1964 researchers at Institut National de la Recherche Agronpmiqeu showed that the skeleton of calves could not develop when magnesium was removed from the diet. Restoring magnesium improved skeletal development and stimulated weight gain.

Animals denied magnesium developed tetany or spasmophilia (abnormal tendency to convulsions; abnormal sensitivity of motor nerves to stimulation with a resultant tendency to spasm.) Subsequent studies of spasmophilia by Dr. L. Bertand showed that a lack of magnesium caused the condition to develop in more than 80 subjects due to hypocalcemia. He also proved that administering calcium did not improve calcemia. However, magnesium improved calcemia and eliminated the condition.

One of the most often referenced studies involving magnesium was conducted by Dr. Guy Abraham and H. Grewel. They worked with a group of postmenopausal women. Those who took a supplement showed significant improvement of bone mass. The supplement contained 500 mg of calcium citrate and 600 mg of magnesium. It also contained vitamin C, 10 B vitamins, vitamin A, vitamin E, vitamin D3, zinc, iron, copper, manganese, boron, iodine, selenium, chromium and other nutrients. There was a modest improvement among the women who did not take the supplement because all of the subjects were given some dietary restrictions: (1) avoid processed foods, (2) limit animal protein and (3) limit refined sugar, salt, alcohol, coffee, tea, chocolate and tobacco. These dietary restrictions could improve the health of millions of people, especially those who are experiencing excessive bone loss. The only thing not on the list was soda and it should have been among the items restricted for bone health.

One test for magnesium involves giving people a dose of the mineral intravenously. Their urine is examined to see how much passes through the body. If the body retains the magnesium, it shows the person to be deficient. In one test of 19 women, 16 retained 90% of the magnesium. These women were also found to have abnormal calcium crystal formations in their bones. In other words, while they had adequate bone mass, their bones were weak or crumbly and subject to break. It is clear that many of the people with good BMD readings who suffer osteoporotic bone breaks have a magnesium deficiency. 50% of the magnesium in the body is in the bones. Magnesium provides strength in the bone matrix.

Many nutritional researchers, who think the current RDA for calcium is too high, also think that the abundance of calcium from dairy products, fortified foods and dietary supplements may actually be contributing to the development of osteoporosis because it causes the loss of magnesium and increases the probability of deficiency.

Magnesium is quickly removed from productive farm land. It is not replaced by the chemical fertilizers normally used. Magnesium content of food in enhanced by adding limestone to farm or garden soil. Most food is grown in magnesium deficient soil. Most foods are harvested before they fully ripen or mature, reducing the content of all minerals including magnesium. Most foods are processed virtually eliminating the small amount of magnesium that may have been in the raw product. The lack of magnesium in the diet contributes to most of the metabolic conditions that dominate and burden our health care system today. Not only bone mass; but also obesity, diabetes and heart conditions would all benefit from an enrichment of magnesium.

POTASSIUM

K + H = Ca

The available literature indicates that potassium plays a minor but direct role in the formulation of bone. It is very important for conserving bone mass and preventing falls that could result in a bone break. A deficiency of potassium can lead to a condition known as *postural hypotension.* It is the opposite of hypertension or high blood pressure. In cases of postural hypotension a person becomes dizzy from the sudden drop in blood pressure. This can lead to a serious fall. Research has shown that people with no known medical cause for this condition are low in potassium. Nearly 25% of those over seventy-five years of age show low blood pressure immediately after standing from a seated or reclined position.

Potassium also plays a role in protective bone mass when it is biologically converted to calcium from the addition of hydrogen. When the blood pH, potential for hydrogen, begins to become acidic, the body can take the excess hydrogen and convert it to calcium as an alkalizing agent. If the body can convert available potassium, it does not have to leech calcium from skeletal bone. The surrender of bone mass as an alkalizing agent is a primary cause of osteoporosis. This condition is caused by the high acid from processed foods and beverages such as carbonated sodas.

Potassium plays a much larger role in cardiovascular health. It has a direct relationship with sodium and kidney function. While potassium and hydrogen can be combined to make calcium carbonate as an alkalizing agent, it is not used by the body in the production of bone mass, calcium hydroxyapatite. According to Kervran only magnesium with stable isotopes of oxygen can make the heavier atoms of calcium used in the osteoblasts that nourish the bones. He also favors calcium transmuted from silica with the addition of carbon..

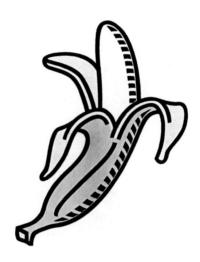

BORON

Arabian physicians used boron as a medicine more than a thousand years ago. As an element it is fifth on the periodic table. It is most commonly used as a cleaning agent in the form of borax. I am sure I am not the only one who remembers Ronald Regan in western attire on black and white television sponsored by Twenty Mule Team Borax. We find borax in our laundry, our toothpaste and our water softener. It is in enamel and glass also. Recent studies have shown boron to be an essential nutrient.

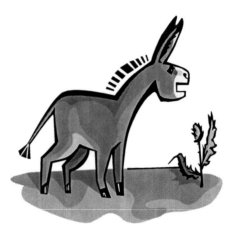

A deficiency of boron in soil can lead to a number of conditions harmful to vegetation. "Cork spot" in apples, "top sickness" in tobacco, "heart-rot" in sugar beets and turnips are among the conditions that occur from a lack of boron in farm soil.

It is known to be supportive to the connective tissues in our joints. Many physicians are using it successfully to treat arthritis. Boron is emerging as an important element for hormonal balance and bone health. Until 1981 boron was not considered important for animals or humans. Forest Nielsen, a biochemist at the Human Nutrition Research Center of the U.S. Department of Agriculture found that a diet deficient in boron and vitamin D caused growth retardation and abnormalities in bone formation. Additional studies showed that requirement for boron was increased if the subject was low in magnesium.

Just to give you a quick review: processed foods from factory farms are low in magnesium content, and most diets are low in boron as well. As it turns out boron enhances the process of hydroxylation in the body. That is the mixing of organic compounds in the body to make hormones and other substances needed for balance and health. It is hydroxylation that produces estrogen and testosterone. It is also the process that converts vitamin D to its active form. Although boron has been recognized as valuable to animal organisms for a relatively short period, even a lay person can quickly recognize its importance to bone health.

One of the primary causes of bone loss among post menopausal women is the unstable stores of estrogen. The treatment of choice for many years was horse estrogen in the form of HRT, Hormone Replacement Therapy. Nielsen and his coworkers discovered that women who had stable intake of boron also had normal levels of estrogen. Apparently, the boron enhanced the hodroxyl production of the hormone when the theca of the ovaries shut down. Nielsen also found that having adequate intake of boron reduced the excretion of both calcium and magnesium in the urine of the subjects.

Here is a trace element that has been around from the beginning that we have only begun to study. What we do know is that it helps convert vitamin D to the active form that is important for forming new bone mass. At the same time, it enhances the production of the reproductive hormones that influence bone mass. Boron is emerging as an important nutrient for our health, especially as it relates to bone mass. Nielsen estimated the daily need for boron at 1 to 2 mg per day. Most people who supplement boron take 3 mg per day.

One might think that in the nearly thirty years that have transpired since Nielsen showed the importance of boron to so many aspects of human health and agriculture that scores of studies would have been carried out to unravel the mysteries of this element. The fact that there have been virtually no studies proves that the incentive for research is profit and health is only a minor consideration. There is little promise for profits from a mineral that is easily mined by the ton and ingested at a rate of 3 mg. There is less chance a court recognize borax as "intellectual property".

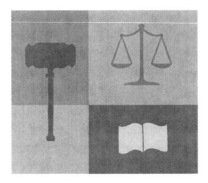

STRONTIUM

I always think of strontium as something Superman
might take for a cold or to regain strength after an
encounter with a dangerous villain. Actually it is a very
common and plentiful element. The space-age sounding
name actually comes from the Scottish village where it
was discovered in 1808, Strontian. It is more plentiful
than carbon in the Earth's

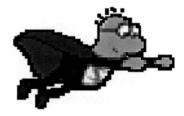

crust. It appears just below calcium on the periodic table.
In fact, it is so close to calcium that it competes with
calcium for absorption in the diet. The limited testing
that has been done on strontium and bone health
indicates that it might be interchangeable with calcium.
There is also the possibility that its closeness to calcium
makes biological transmutation an easy maneuver in
living matter.

The U.S. Navy examined the teeth of 270,000 recruits
and found that only 360 of them were completely free of
cavities. Of the 360, 10% were from an area of Ohio
where the water contains an above normal amount of
strontium. Subsequent animal studies showed that
administering strontium reduced the incidence of tooth
decay.

Clinical trials have shown a positive relationship between bone mass and strontium since the 1940s. In 1959 the Mayo Clinic tested strontium on thirty two people diagnosed with osteoporosis. They were given 1.7 grams of strontium lactate daily. 84% reported marked relief from bone pain, the remaining 16% reported moderate relief. Unfortunately, pain is too subjective for a scientific conclusion. The study took place before the development of the modern MBD tests, but X-rays showed improved bone mass among 78% of the subjects. Not much was done with the findings, and the radio active strontium scare of the 50s caused the element to fall out of favor for human use.

Later it was shown that radioactive strontium can be removed from the body by administering stable forms of the same element. As far as safety is concerned, it would not have taken much research to find strontium listed in *Squire's Companion to the British Pharmacopeia* 1884. No dangerous side effects were experienced. As late as 1955 strontium was listed in the *Dispensary of the United States* at dose levels as high as 400 mg per day with no toxic results. Again, a substance that is mined by the ton and used in milligrams has little appeal for the pharmaceutical researchers whose mission is developing patents on substances that manage diseases, not cure them.

The link between strontium and healthy bone mass may not be clearly defined, but it cannot be denied based on the limited investigations that have been carried out. In one three year study of 5,091 postmenopausal women those taking strontium along with calcium and vitamin D were able to avoid 41% of the hip fractures experienced by those taking only the calcium and vitamin D. Another similar study involved 1,649 post-menopausal women. Those taking only calcium and vitamin D showed a 1.3% loss of bone in the lower spine when given a BMD test. Those who also took 680 mg of strontium increased bone mass by 14.4% in the lower spine and 8.3% in the large bone at the top of the thigh.

From these tests and others we have learned that strontium reduces bone loss or resorption, and at the same time it increases the formation of new bone. Apparently strontium causes osteoblasts to form and multiply. While the exact pathways may not be defined, bone tissue cultures exposed to strontium synthesized more bone matrix and new collagen.

If strontium enhances the work of calcium and vitamin D, why do we not put it in our calcium supplements? Because strontium competes with calcium for absorption and both would be reduced by putting them together. Strontium works best taken alone, several hours before or after the calcium rich foods or supplements.

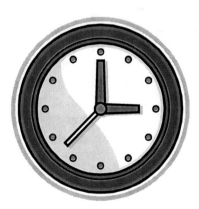

SILICA

Si + C = Ca

Natural healers throughout the ages have used the herb, horsetail (Equisetum), to treat broken bones. Studies have shown that silica is involved in the early stages of calcification. According to Krevran, in its elemental form silica or silicon can cause decalcification, but organic silica causes calcification. It is important for connective tissue and for the formation of the collagen needed for healthy bone mass.

Chicks fed a diet deficient in silica experienced significant bone deformities. When silica was added to their diet their growth rate increased by 50% and their skeletons became normal. In another animal study the subjects developed highly abnormal skulls leading investigators to conclude silica is needed for the development of soft bone, including cartilage and connective tissue.

When silica is removed from the diet there is a loss of calcium from the bone. When silica is returned to the diet, calcium returns to the bone. Researchers have determined that when a baby chick is hatching in an egg, the calcium used to form its skeleton does not come from the shell. When the chick hatches the calcium content of the shell remains the same. The calcium content of the hatching egg begins to increase on the tenth day of incubation. The membrane between the shell and the white and yoke, however, is rich in silica. This silica is biologically transmuted into calcium as the chick forms its skeleton.

Other studies of laying hens have shown that without silica in the diet the eggs do not have healthy shells.

In addition to helping the human body heal a broken bone, horsetail also supports the development of healthy hair, skin and nails. It has been used successfully in the treatment of tuberculosis. In 1846 Pierre Jousset, a master homoeopathist, delivered a thesis showing that horsetail could speed the calcification of lung caverns and thus speed the healing of patients with tuberculosis.

Simply stated, if silica is needed for collagen, and collagen is needed for bone health, silica is an important nutrient. The Spring horsetail contains the most silica. Here again there is little hope for meaningful medical examination of silica. As an extract from a common weed, there is little chance of getting a patent. It also remains an inexpensive and effective nutrient for avoiding bone loss.

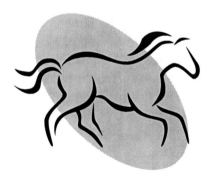

ZINC

Zinc is found in every cell of the human body. Perhaps, the statement should read "zinc is found in every healthy cell of a human body". A zinc deficiency can lead to a host of problems including anemia, low immune response, poor wound healing, sexual dysfunction, dermatitis and retarded growth. Because so many foods in the American diet are processed, particularly sugar and white flour, most people are low in zinc. One study found that 68% of adults were getting less than two-thirds of the RDA of 15 mg. Zinc is necessary for the synthesis of protein and DNA. Without adequate zinc the body struggles to produce the osteoblasts and osteoclasts needed for maintaining healthy bone mass.

The evidence suggests that a zinc deficiency can contribute to the development of osteoporosis. One study of elderly individuals, 60 to 80 years of age, found that 90% were low in zinc and most not only had bone loss, but also low immune function. Another study of people with bone loss of the bone that holds the lower teeth, the alveolar ridge of the mandible, were low in dietary zinc. Many studies have shown that zinc is important for bone health. With its effect on so many body functions it should not be surprising that zinc is an important nutrient for bone health. Zinc can even enhance sexual function and for that reason oysters are often considered an aphrodisiac.

MANGANESE

Manganese has been shown in animal studies and limited human studies to play an important role in bone health. A manganese deficiency is known to cause bone deformity and other serious conditions including challenges to the pancreas and insulin production. Manganese is needed for the formation of compounds called mucopolysaccharides that provide a structure on which calcification can take place.

Rats given a manganese deficient diet had a reduction in calcification of the femur and thinner than normal bones. In the same studies the bones were more prone to break from physical trauma.

In 1963 after a decade of research Pierre Baranger verified that during the germination of leguminous seeds manganese disappeared and was replaced by iron. This established a relationship between manganese and iron. Both are helpful in delivering oxygen. Kervran believes that we should supplement manganese for iron in the human body, because the living tissue biologically transmutes manganese to organic iron without the harmful side effects experienced by those who take Ferris sulfate.

Manganese is plentiful in mustard greens, kale and chard. It is also found in brown rice and most beans. Processed foods can lose almost all of their manganese content.

PHOSPHORUS

Phosphorus is the second most abundant mineral in the human body, right behind calcium. The two elements work closely in building and maintaining healthy bones and teeth. 85% of the phosphorus is found in teeth and bones and about 10% circulates in the blood stream. The remaining 5% is of major importance. Phosphorus is a prime component of nucleic acid, the substance that supports RNA/DNA. In this capacity phosphorus supports cell development and healthy growth. It is an important element for energy because it participates in the breakdown of carbohydrates, fats and proteins. In the kidneys, it helps filter waste materials from the blood.

While the modern American diet tends to reduce the amount of important elements we get from our food, phosphorus remains abundant and getting too much is more common than having a deficiency. Too much phosphorus leads to calcification or hardening of the organs and arteries. Excessive phosphorus also interferes with the balance of iron, calcium, magnesium and zinc. The body releases calcium from the stores in the skeleton to balance the excessive phosphorus. For example meat and poultry contain ten times more phosphorus than calcium. A single serving of soda contains 500mg of phosphorus. High intake of phosphorus is a leading contributor to osteoporosis and poor dental health. While a phosphorus deficiency may be rare, it can be serious. Bone pain and fragility, stiff and painful joints, numbness, irregular breathing, fatigue, weakness and irritability can be caused by reduced phosphorus. The leading cause of depleted phosphorus is exposure to aluminum, especially from the use of some antacids. A delicate balance between calcium and phosphorus is necessary for maintaining healthy bone mass.

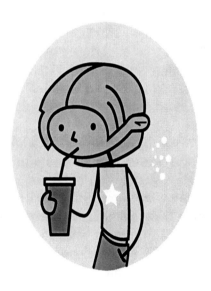

VITAMIN D

The sunshine vitamin is emerging as a primary component of healthy bone mass. When converted by the body to its active form, it is a hormone that supports the recalcification of healthy bone. We can get a limited amount of vitamin D from our diet; it is in fish and fish oils. Synthetic forms are added to milk and some dairy products, but these synthetic forms have been shown to be less bioavailable and their content can vary greatly from product to product. The most consistent source of vitamin D remains the sun. In sunlight our bodies convert cholesterol to vitamin D. There are scores of studies supporting the importance of vitamin D for bone health. Scores more studies show it to be vital for immune response, cancer protection, inflammatory bowel diseases, and many other body functions.

Patients with osteoporosis invariably test low for vitamin D. Lifestyle can limit this important vitamin for many people. Less time outdoors, sunscreen products and geography are some of the environmental reasons for vitamin D deficiency. We need only a few minutes in the sun several times per week to produce the needed amount of vitamin D. In some parts of the world however, the amount of sunshine is limited during the winter seasons. For people living north or south of the equator by more than 40 degrees there is a greater risk for osteoporosis and other conditions related to vitamin D deficiency.

Dr William Grant, an independent researcher from Virginia, has examined the difference in cancer rates based on where people live. Using data from the Atlas of Cancer Mortality, he found death rates from breast, colon and ovarian cancers in Boston and New England were almost twice as high as they were in the southwest from 1950 to 1994.

He found the same link, with varying increased risk, for 13 cancers including bladder, kidney, stomach and non-Hodgkin's lymphoma. In an interview with the BBC Grant estimated that at least 25% of the breast cancers in the U.K. were caused by a deficiency of vitamin D.

Using sunscreen products with an SPF of 8 will reduce vitamin D production by 95%. Women who cover their bodies for religious or cultural reasons are more likely to test low for vitamin D. People with darker skin pigment need more sun exposure than those with lighter skin pigment to produce the needed amount of vitamin D.

Supplementing vitamin D seems prudent. Most nutrition oriented practitioners are suggesting 1000 iu per day, and in some cases higher amounts are indicated. There is broad consensus that the RDA is much too low. Currently the RDA ranges from 200 iu for those under fifty years of age to 400 iu for over fifty and 600 iu for those over seventy. The recommendations on the cutting edge of emerging science would at least double the current RDA.

Much of the vitamin D deficiency can be traced to a modern-day fear of the sun. We are constantly reminded by everybody from the TV weather people to the clerks at the cosmetic counters to "wear sunscreen". Dr. Michael Holick, a professor at Boston College has been a leader in urging limited sun exposure to increase the availability of vitamin D. He suggests avoiding the sun during its brightest hours during the middle part of the day, but getting sun a few minutes at a time several times a week. Several articles in

113

respected journals have withdrawn from the emphasis on sunscreen in favor of the need for vitamin D. Obviously, the corporate-mindset would have us buy sunscreen and buy vitamin D supplements to offset the lack of the vitamin that results from the use of the sunscreen. Win win for them, lose lose for us. After all, sunshine is free. There must be a proper balance between sun exposure and protection from the cancer causing rays. Otherwise, we have people getting cancer from a lack of vitamin D while others are getting cancer because they are in the sun to get vitamin D.

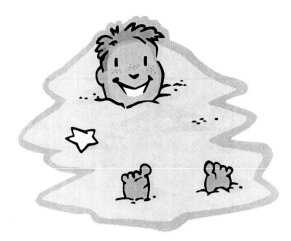

VITAMIN C

Vitamin C is needed for the synthesis of collagen. Without collagen our bones would be brittle and more prone to breakage. Several recent studies have shown that vitamin C can help build and maintain bone mass. In one study with mice osteoporosis was induced by restricting vitamin C intake. Most elderly test low for vitamin C. Even those who eat diets containing vitamin C rich foods and those who supplement can test low. For some reason the human body does not store vitamin C and the only reserve is the surplus at any given time. Studies show that people who take the mega-doses of vitamin C in the morning, may be low on it later in the day. Apparently what the body is not using at any given time is being processed through the kidneys and flushed out. In fact the only people cautioned not to take large doses of vitamin C are those who have limited kidney function. They are advised to take no more than 100 mg per day.

As an antioxidant vitamin C is believed to inhibit the cytokines that are present during bone loss. Antioxidants can also protect the bones from oxidative stress. NAC, N-acytle cysteine, and vitamin E have been shown to protect bone mass. Professor Tim Chambers and colleagues at St. George's Hospital Medical School at the University of London found a link between vitamin C and estrogen. Writing in the *Journal of Clinical Investigation* they showed that giving mice 20 mg of vitamin C daily prevented bone loss after inducing menopause by ovariectomy. Chambers wrote,

"I believe that our results have revealed the mechanism through which estrogen protects bone against osteoporosis. It should be possible in the future to prevent osteoporosis in postmenopausal women by giving them antioxidants".

Older studies have shown that vitamin C contributes to bone density by improving the markers of bone turnover. Remember it is normal to lose bone mass as we leech calcium and other minerals into our blood stream. Osteoporosis occurs when we do not replace, or regenerate the bone mass that we are losing. There is some evidence that indicates that taking large doses of vitamin C will not protect the body over a period of several hours and that smaller more frequent doses may be more effective. One theory concerning our inability to store vitamin C is that when we were foraging we were getting a continuous supply of the vitamin and our bodies did not develop a capacity to store it or make it.

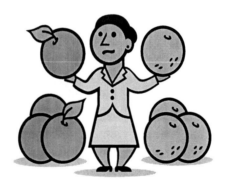

VITAMIN K

Vitamin K is a fat soluble vitamin that can be produced by our gut flora or obtained from green leafy vegetables in our diet. The "K" comes from the German word "koagulation". Coagulation refers to the clotting of blood, or the process that helps the body stop bleeding when a wound has flushed or cleansed itself. Clotting becomes a problem when a person is taking a blood thinning medication, and the consumption of foods containing vitamin K may be restricted. Vitamin K is a cofactor for an enzyme that catalyzes the carboxylation of the amino acid glutamine into a protein needed for binding calcium. This protein is a component of the osteoblasts that rebuild bone. Not all vitamin K comes from diet. Actually, the more active form of the vitamin involved in production of osteoblasts, is made by our digestive bacteria.

Studies have demonstrated a clear relationship between vitamin K and age-related bone loss or osteoporosis. In the Nurses' Health Study that followed more than 72,000 women for a period of ten years the risk of hip fracture was highest among those with the lowest intakes of the vitamin. In the Framingham Heart Study that followed over 800 elderly men and women for seven years, those in the top 25% in consumption of vitamin K were at lower risk for hip fracture by 65%. At the same time investigators found no association between vitamin K and bone mineral density, BMD, nor was there an association between BMD and bone break. These findings indicate strong bone is not always assured by density.

Studies that measured the levels of osteocalcin, a bone-related protein that is carried in the blood stream and known to be a sensitive marker for bone formation, showed a direct relationship to risk for fracture. One study of 195 institutionalized women over the age of seventy were six times more likely to experience bone break because they were low in osteocalcin. Another study of 7,500 elderly women living independently with high levels of osteocalcin were found less likely to experience bone break from osteoporosis. While vitamin K is essential for the synthesis of osteocalcin, supplementation with vitamin D can also increase its blood levels. It was concluded that circulating levels of osteocalcin could be a marker for the quality of the diet. The subjects may not be getting enough green leafy vegetables or protein. Circulating levels of osteocalcin could also reflect the health of the gut flora and the ability to synthesize the vitamin in the digestive process.

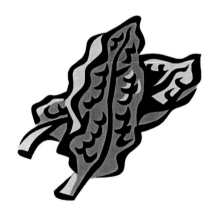

"Pleasant words are as an honeycomb, sweet to the soul and health to the bones."

Proverbs 16:24

NUTRITION TO AVOID OSTEOPOROSIS

I truly hope that I have not depressed you with the information presented above. If I have, I certainly hope you will not shoot the messenger. There is a brighter side that I want to leave with you. The human body is a mystery of systems and organization. Its workings have been evolving for a long time. As long as we are alive we are constantly evolving or becoming. Becoming is our journey. Developing is our mission. As long as we have breath we can regenerate. Air, water, sunlight, rest and proper food can give us the elements we need to recover and maintain. Love and gratitude can energize the process. When we stop evolving we reach equilibrium and it is over, our work is done. In the meantime, despite toxic chemicals, adulterated agriculture and all the other things I have been writing about, given half a chance the human body can maintain balance and health. The question then is how do we give it half a chance?

Get plenty of fresh air. Stretch and breathe deeply several times each day. Raising your arms and filling your lungs with fresh air stimulates the production of vitamins and improves digestion and elimination. You have heard that *we are what we eat.* Unfortunately, we are also what we have not eliminated. How long would the motor in your car be able to run without an exhaust system? How long can the body function if it carries around a couple of days of used food? You have heard about the importance of location, location, location. Consider the importance of elimination, elimination, elimination. It is amazing how many conditions can be cleared up with improved elimination. Fresh air and simple exercise can help.

Water is also important. We all have different needs for hydration that change daily depending on what we consume and our body functions. There are formulas, such as 8 oz of water for every twenty pounds of body weight, which can be used to determine the daily goals for water intake. There is also the blanket directive that would have everybody drink 8 glasses per day. There are no conclusive studies on how much water we need. It is my anecdotal experience that people who do not drink enough pure water, not just liquids, have problems eliminating. Many appear to have other problems that could be explained by dehydration. I have seen people cure themselves of everything from depression to skin conditions by increasing their water intake. I have also seen people who may have over challenged their kidneys with excessive water consumption. We all have to find our happy medium and make sure we have adequate water for our bodies to function properly.

We need sunlight. In addition to the basic need for the production of vitamin D, we need the sun for many other functions in the body. Our endocrines need sunlight. We have many receptors for light in our eyes that have nothing to do with sight, but carry stimulation to the brain. There is a cascade of hormonal activity triggered by sunlight. Many of us have drifted into a lifestyle that does not provide the sunlight needed by the body for proper function. Many also have become so fearful of the sun that they cover their bodies with clothing or sunscreen lotions. If we are going to get off an airplane from a frigid climate to spend a few days on a tropical beach, we need protection. If we are out in the noon day sun, we might need protection. But taking a walk in the early morning or late afternoon a few times per week without sun glasses or sunscreens can give our bodies the exposure needed for proper function.

One of the biggest challenges to health and well-being today is adequate rest. Our electrified lifestyle allows us to be occupied with work and pleasure long after the sun goes down, or long before it comes up. Do you know anybody who is not "burning the candle at both ends"? We push our children and ourselves during too many hours of the day. We create stress, sometimes for all the wrong reasons. We become overly occupied with seeking control of our lives through goals and standards of our own design. We have lost the courage needed to allow life to come, or to take it as it does come. Prayer and meditation are not effective while multi-tasking. When we learn to live our lives as spiritual beings, we find harmony in all things.

Our bodies are about 6 and 1/3 pounds of earthly elements and the rest is seawater or saline. Take away the energy of the spirit of life and you have a sack of seawater that will evaporate to leave 6 1/3 pounds of dust. While we are still evolving and becoming, it is our food that bonds our bodies with the earth, or replenishes the elements of the earth. Food is the bonding agent of life. It renews our relationship with the Earthly Mother and it bonds us with those with whom we share our food, our family and our friends. The Old Testament teaches that a *meal with friends is the reward of our labors under the sun.* Obviously, the food will do more to sustain our bodies if it comes to our table free of chemicals and adulteration. It also serves us better if it comes from the earth near where we live. We should try to eat local and in season. We should prepare our food in a way that will honor the earth and our bodies. We should also set our tables with love and honor the bonding that is to come with the meal. If we are eating local and in season, we will most likely have the needed fiber in our food to avoid problems of elimination. Processing not only destroys nutrition, it also limits the fiber. If we are going to turn the tide of metabolic illness in our lives, we will begin by supporting local food production. We must also honor the microbes that make our life possible. The microbes that make the Earth fertile to grow good food, and the microbes in our digestive and elimination tracts. Without them the soil is infirmed and so are our bodies. In the section on Our Hidden Symbiots I tried to demonstrate the importance of the good bacteria that support our life experience. If we do not have healthy gut flora, we do not have health. These bacteria work with our digestive enzymes to prepare the food for us to metabolize. They even synthesize some of the vitamins we need. Without them our food is not easily metabolized and assimilated. As long as we are metabolizing, we are evolving and becoming. The more efficient we are at metabolizing the more effective we are in what we will become. Do not be afraid of the forces of greed that are distorting our world. When we surrender to faith, we have control of our lives without fear.

The Maya or "corn people" cultivated corn 9,000 years ago while the Chinese were planting soy. These people knew two things about the Sun: that it controls fertility, and that it is the supreme energy source. Perhaps we should rediscover these facts of our Universe before

122

this politically and commercially corrupt fossil fueled charade engulfing us increases the Gulf of Mexico "lifeless" zone from the size of New Jersey to include New York, Pennsylvania and New England. It will grow larger each year, as long as we ignore the Sun and *sustainable, organic farming.* Can we produce enough food without synthetic nitrogen? Yes! However, we will have to cooperate with the natural microbes that liberate nitrogen. We will have to cooperate with nature and live in the world that evolved with Intelligence. We will have to give up our greed and vanity-driven belief that we can make a better world than the one we have been given. We will have to stop creating chaos out of harmony. The natural way of doing things makes us independent and free. It is fear and dependence that build empires and amass wealth. Fear and dependence take away our freedom to be and become.

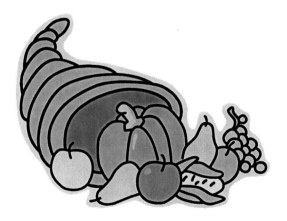

RESOURCES AND REFERENCES

The China Study, T. Colin Campbell, PhD and Thomas Campbell II, BenBella Book, Inc

Fats That Heal, Fats That Kill, Udo Erasmus, Alive Books

Subatomic Physics, Ernest M Henley and Alejandro Garcia, World Scientific, Inc

Riddled With Life, Marlene Zuk ,Harcourt, Inc

Good Germs, Bad Germs, Jessica Snyder Sachs, Hill and Wang

The Genius Within, Frank T. Verstosick, Jr M.D., Harcourt

Biological Transmutations, Louis C. Kervran, Swan House Publishing, Co

Genetic Routette. Jeffrey M. Smith, Yes Books

Principles of Modern Microbiology, Mark Wheelis, Jones and Bartlett

Microbiology, Principles and Explorations, Jacquelyn G Black, Wiley

The Amber Waves of Gain, How the Government Makes Us Fat, Gene Ladd, Pleasant Stone Farm, Ltd

Fatal Harvest. Various contributors, Island Press

Preventing and Reversing Osteoporosis, Alan R. Gaby, M.D., Three Rivers Press

The Myth of Osteoporosis, Gillian Sanson, MCD Century Publications, LLC

Journal of Reproductive Medicine 35, 1990, Abraham and Grewal, Magnesium

Harvard School of Public Health, The Nurses Study

www.blessmybones.com

www.nih.gov, The Women's Health Initiative

www.wellbeingjournal.com for related articles

www.organicconsumers.com for information on health food

www.responsibletechnology.org for information on Genetic Modification

www.ucsusa.org for the Union of Concerned Scientists

www.nof.org National Osteoporosis Foundation

www.nlm.nih.gov/medlineplus/osteoporosis.html MedLine Plus information center

www.mayoclinic.com/health/osteoporosis/ Treatments and research at the Mayo Clinic

http://www.medicinenet.com/osteoporosis/article.htm Information Center

2045788

Made in the USA